* * * * * *

'Fun graphic book bringing dyspraxia … ple activities offer support fo… 's book also shows just …

– Alison Patrick, au…
We are th…

'Having this book at 13, whe… PE I was yelled at not only by teammates, but … teachers too, would've been life changing. But the next best thing is having it now! This book is the hug all dyspraxic young people need.'

– Meg, creator of *I'm Autistic, Now What?* (YouTube)

'A delightful, much-needed book about something that's much under-recognized. Full of warmth, humour and hope, *A Trip into a Dyspraxic Person's World* is an essential read for young dyspraxics who are looking to understand themselves better. Or for older dyspraxics who wish they'd had this kind of understanding when they were young.'

– Maxine Roper, author of *No Heels, No Problem: A Neurodivergent Survival Guide to Adult Life when you are Dyspraxic or ADHD*

'*A Trip into a Dyspraxic Person's World* is an unapologetic glimpse into what it truly means to live with a dyspraxic mind, while navigating an often-inaccessible world that does not fully understand dyspraxia. Through Lotty O'Neill's engaging illustration style and methods of explaining dyspraxia, dyspraxia feels easy for even the most unfamiliar reader to understand. That's exactly what we need at this very moment, when neurodivergence is still under-supported and misunderstood despite having an increasing amount of mainstream representation.'

– Rosemary Richings, author of *Stumbling through Space and Time: Living Life with Dyspraxia*

'*A Trip into a Dyspraxic Person's World* is a beautifully engaging and relatable read for young people. It explores challenges, strengths, language and co-occurrence through captivating stories, making neurodiversity easy to understand. A must-read that will inspire and enlighten both dyspraxic young people and their peers.'

– Tumi Sotire (The Black Dyspraxic)

* * * * * *

A TRIP INTO A DYSPRAXIC PERSON'S WORLD

of related interest

All About Dyspraxia
Understanding Developmental Coordination Disorder
Kathy Hoopmann
ISBN 978 1 78775 835 3
eISBN 978 1 78775 836 0

We are the Dyspraxia Champions!
The Amazing Talents, Skills and Everyday Life of Children with Dyspraxia
Alison Patrick
Illustrated by Tim Stringer
Foreword by Jonathan Levy
ISBN 978 1 83997 910 1
eISBN 978 1 83997 911 8

Stumbling Through Space and Time
Living Life with Dyspraxia
Rosemary Richings
ISBN 978 1 83997 269 0
eISBN 978 1 83997 270 6

A Trip into a DYSPRAXIC PERSON'S WORLD

LOTTY O'NEILL

Jessica Kingsley Publishers
London and Philadelphia

First published in Great Britain in 2026 by Jessica Kingsley Publishers
An imprint of John Murray Press

1

Front cover image source: Lotty O'Neill.

A CIP catalogue record for this title is available from the British Library and the Library of Congress

ISBN 978 1 83997 517 2

Printed and bound in China by Leo Paper Products Ltd

Jessica Kingsley Publishers' policy is to use papers that are natural, renewable and recyclable products and made from wood grown in sustainable forests. The logging and manufacturing processes are expected to conform to the environmental regulations of the country of origin.

Jessica Kingsley Publishers
Carmelite House
50 Victoria Embankment
London EC4Y ODZ

www.jkp.com

John Murray Press
Part of Hodder & Stoughton Ltd
An Hachette Company

The authorised representative in the EEA is Hachette Ireland,
8 Castlecourt Centre, Dublin 15, D15 XTP3, Ireland (email: info@hbgi.ie)

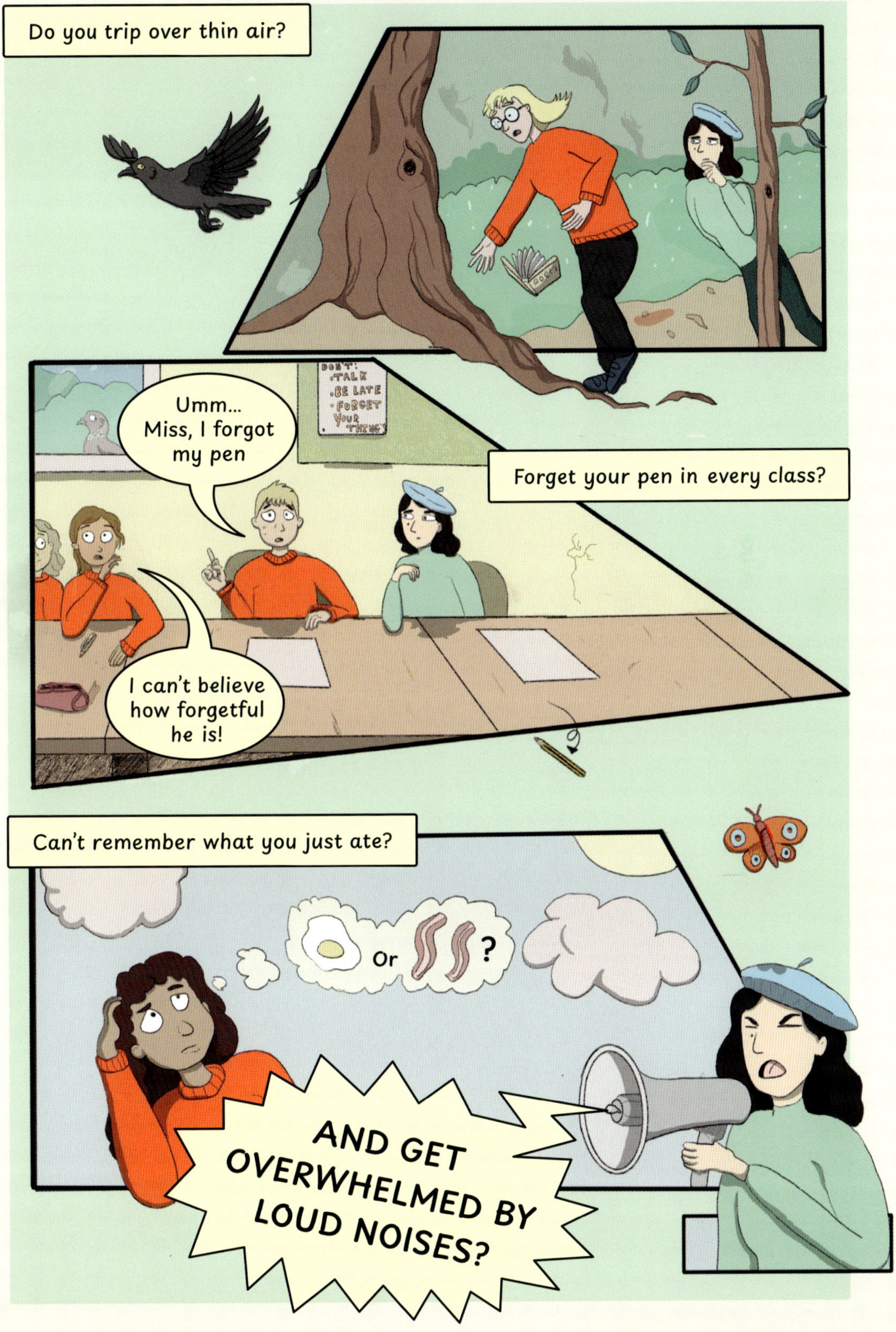
Do you trip over thin air?
Umm... Miss, I forgot my pen
Forget your pen in every class?
I can't believe how forgetful he is!
Can't remember what you just ate?
Or ?
AND GET OVERWHELMED BY LOUD NOISES?

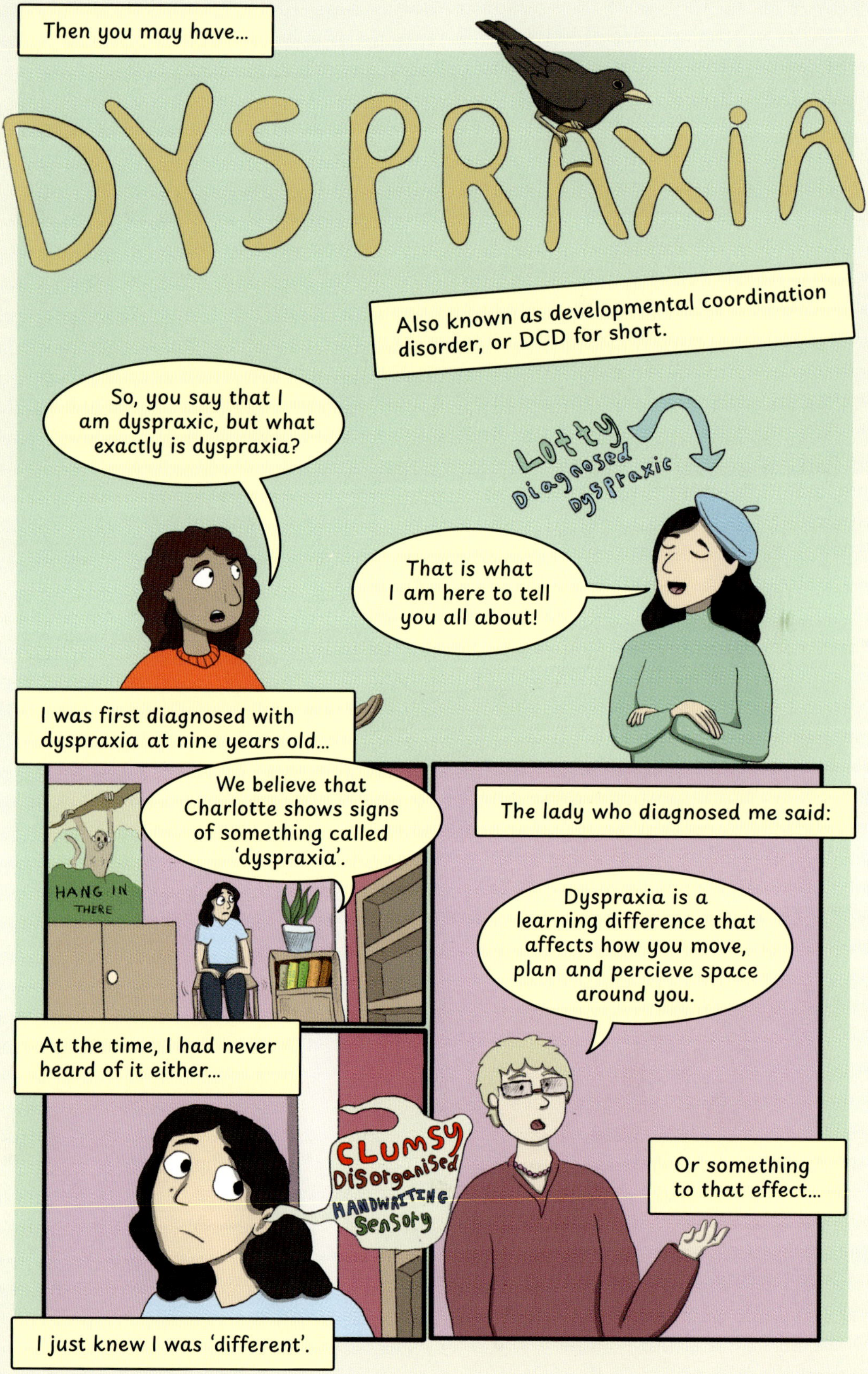

Then you may have...
DYSPRAXIA
Also known as developmental coordination disorder, or DCD for short.
So, you say that I am dyspraxic, but what exactly is dyspraxia?
Lotty
Diagnosed Dyspraxic
That is what I am here to tell you all about!
I was first diagnosed with dyspraxia at nine years old...
HANG IN THERE
We believe that Charlotte shows signs of something called 'dyspraxia'.
At the time, I had never heard of it either...
CLUMSY
DISorganiSed
HANDWRITING
Sensory
I just knew I was 'different'.
The lady who diagnosed me said:
Dyspraxia is a learning difference that affects how you move, plan and percieve space around you.
Or something to that effect...

Hopefully, by the end of this book you will have a good understanding of what dyspraxia is!

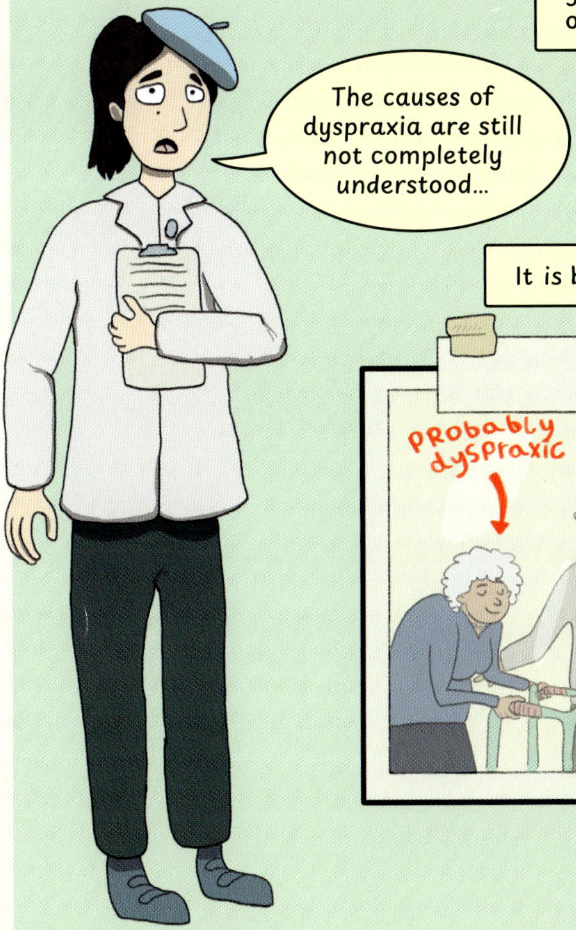

It is believed to run in families,

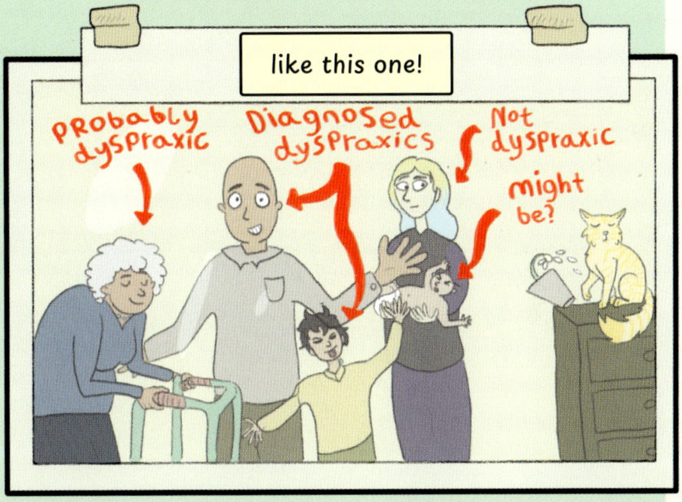

It may be caused by the brain misunderstanding information from the senses.

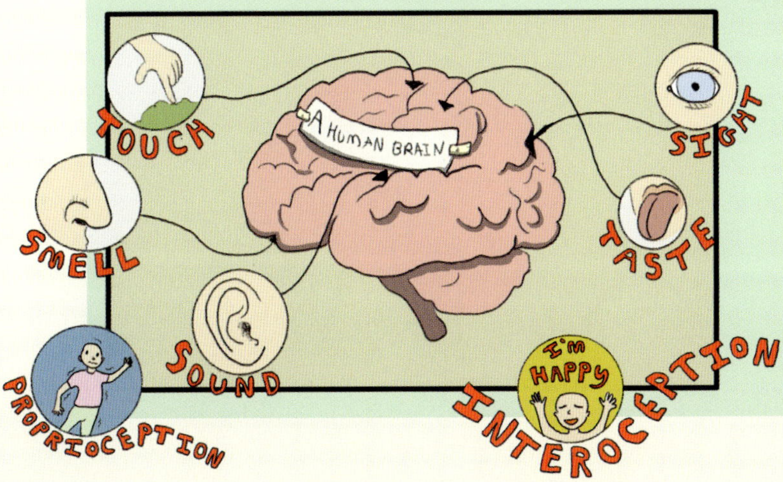

The senses are how we gather information about the world around us through special organs, such as our nose or tongue! These organs send information about what is happening around us to the brain through electrical signals.

Did you know that we have eight senses in total? As well as sight, hearing, smell, taste and touch, we have three less well-known senses: vestibular (balance), proprioception (body awareness) and interoception (how we feel inside).

It may also be caused by the amount of time it takes for cells called neurons to send information from the brain to the rest of the body.

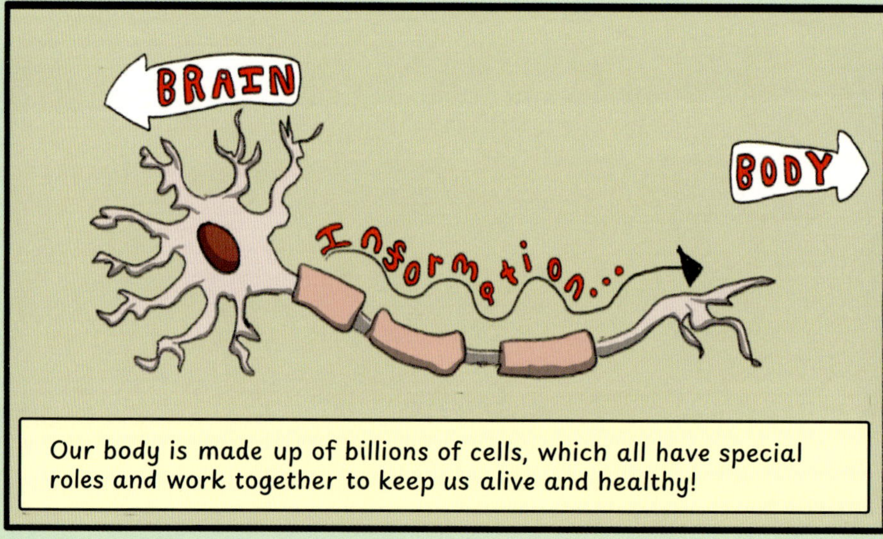

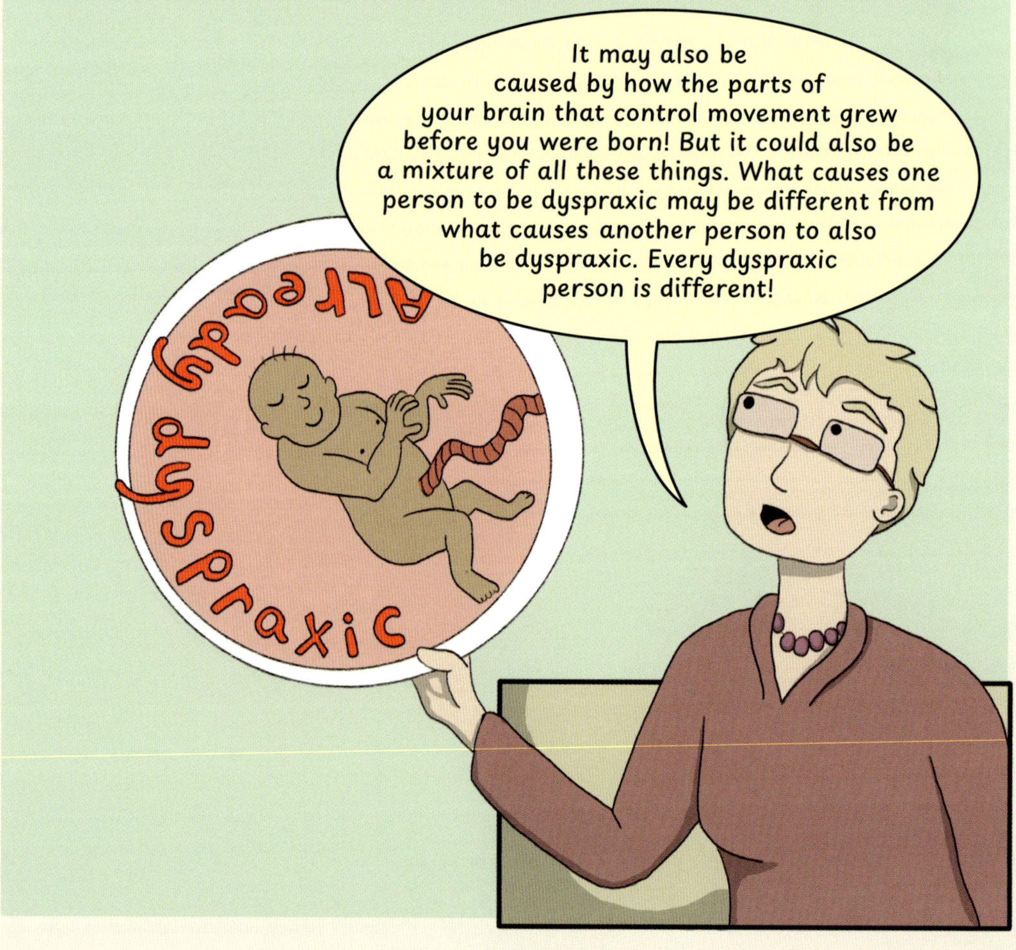
It may also be caused by how the parts of your brain that control movement grew before you were born! But it could also be a mixture of all these things. What causes one person to be dyspraxic may be different from what causes another person to also be dyspraxic. Every dyspraxic person is different!
Already dyspraxic

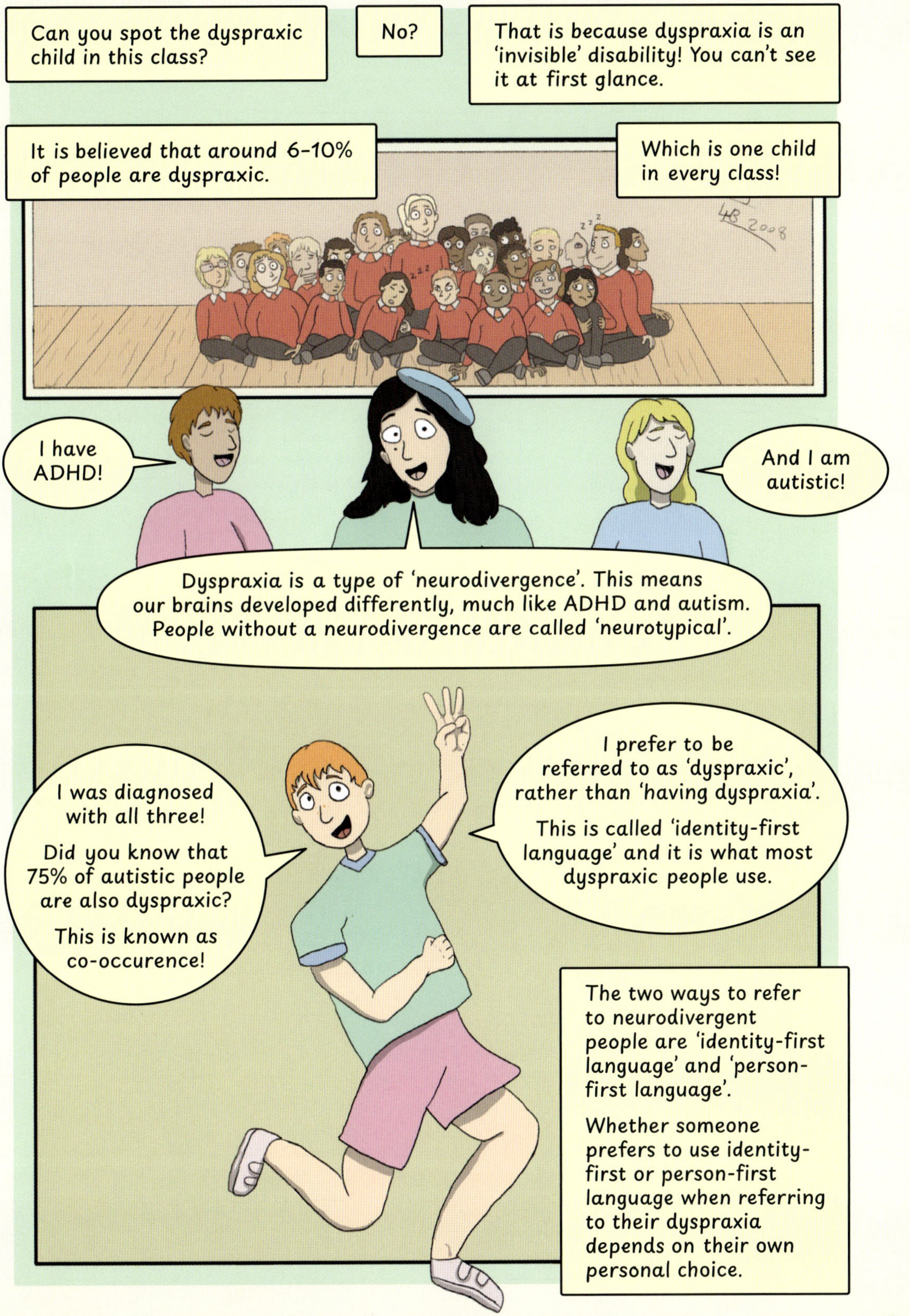

Can you spot the dyspraxic child in this class?
No?
That is because dyspraxia is an 'invisible' disability! You can't see it at first glance.
It is believed that around 6–10% of people are dyspraxic.
Which is one child in every class!
4B 2008
I have ADHD!
And I am autistic!
Dyspraxia is a type of 'neurodivergence'. This means our brains developed differently, much like ADHD and autism. People without a neurodivergence are called 'neurotypical'.
I was diagnosed with all three!
Did you know that 75% of autistic people are also dyspraxic?
This is known as co-occurence!
I prefer to be referred to as 'dyspraxic', rather than 'having dyspraxia'.
This is called 'identity-first language' and it is what most dyspraxic people use.
The two ways to refer to neurodivergent people are 'identity-first language' and 'person-first language'.
Whether someone prefers to use identity-first or person-first language when referring to their dyspraxia depends on their own personal choice.

Identity-first Language

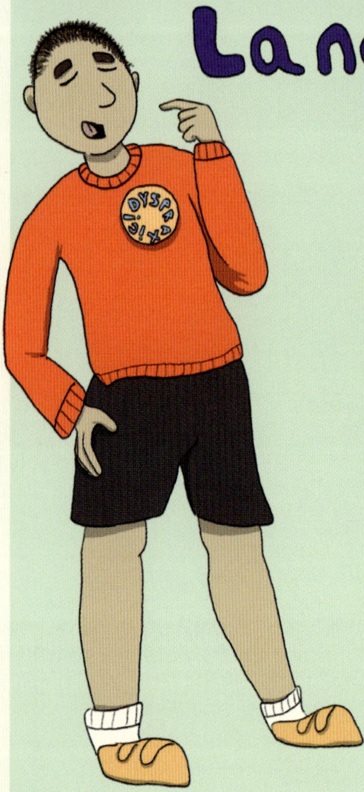

An example of 'identity-first language' is referring to someone as 'dyspraxic'.

The majority of dyspraxic people prefer this, as it makes it clear that their dyspraxia is a part of them, not something that can be removed.

By calling yourself dyspraxic, you can claim it as an identity, which can help with self-acceptance. Dyspraxia is not something that can be cured, and it can also come with plenty of positive aspects.

But this isn't the only way to refer to yourself. I personally use both identity-first and person-first language!

Person-first Language

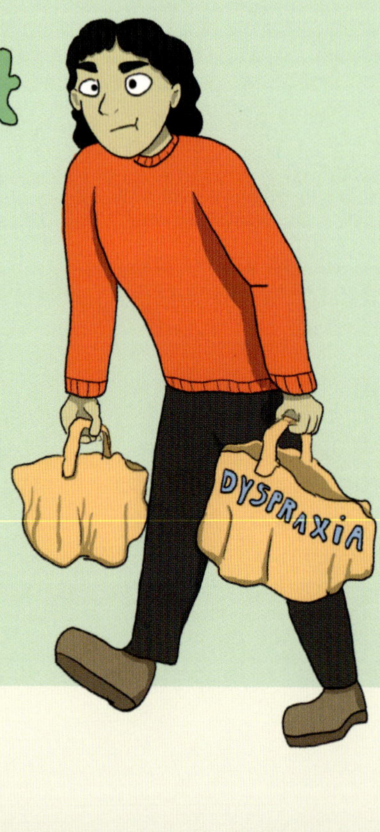

Person-first language is used when you refer to someone or yourself as 'having dyspraxia'. This type of language suggests that dyspraxia is separate from a person.

Many people complain that this sounds like dyspraxia is baggage that can be picked up or put down at any point. This might put more pressure on us to 'overcome our condition', even when that may not be possible.

This language is most commonly used in schools and hospital settings.

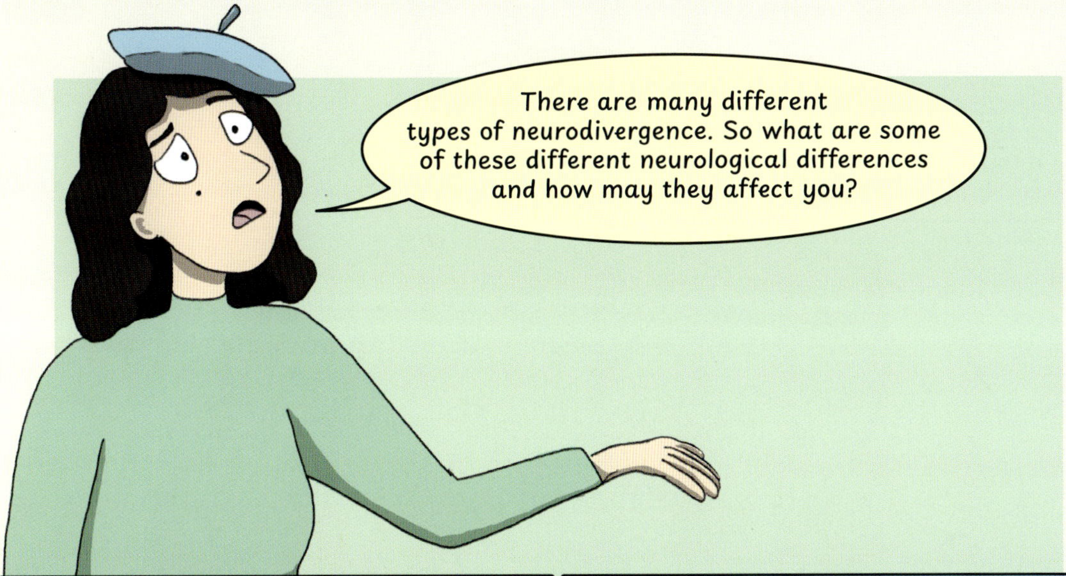
There are many different types of neurodivergence. So what are some of these different neurological differences and how may they affect you?

Autism Spectrum Disorder

- You may struggle to read facial expressions and your face may not show how you are feeling.
- You may make repetitive actions or repeat words, this is known as 'stimming'.
- You may like to have a strict routine.
- You may not speak (something known as 'non-verbal') or you may talk a lot!
- You might get overwhelmed easily.
- You may not make eye contact when speaking to people.
- You may be very good at concentrating.
- You can gain a lot of knowledge about a subject that greatly interests you (also known as a special interest).

ADHD

- You may have difficulty concentrating.
- You may struggle to focus on one task or may be able to hyperfocus on a task.
- You may have a lot of energy that you struggle to express.
- You may have difficulty organizing tasks and be forgetful.
- You may struggle to wait your turn when speaking.
- You may be able to do things at short notice and can be very flexible with your time.
- You have the ability to focus really hard on the things you enjoy. This is called hyperfocus.

Dyscalculia

- You may struggle with mental mathematics and have problems counting.
- You may be unable to read mathematical equations and remember how to repeat them.
- You may find it hard to follow recipes.
- You may have problems following directions.
- You may find yourself struggling to understand graphs and charts.
- You probably have other strengths. For example, you may be a great storyteller or brilliant at football.
- You may find that you are good at speaking and writing!

Dyslexia

- You may confuse words that look similar.
- You may struggle to read.
- You may find it hard to spell words.
- You may write more slowly than other people.
- You may have difficulty telling the difference between left and right.
- You may struggle to follow instructions.
- You may forget dates and names.
- You may be a big picture thinker. This means you can focus on the whole, whilst others focus on the details.
- You may find that you are a creative problem solver.

There are often many similarities between different neurodivergent conditions, such as...

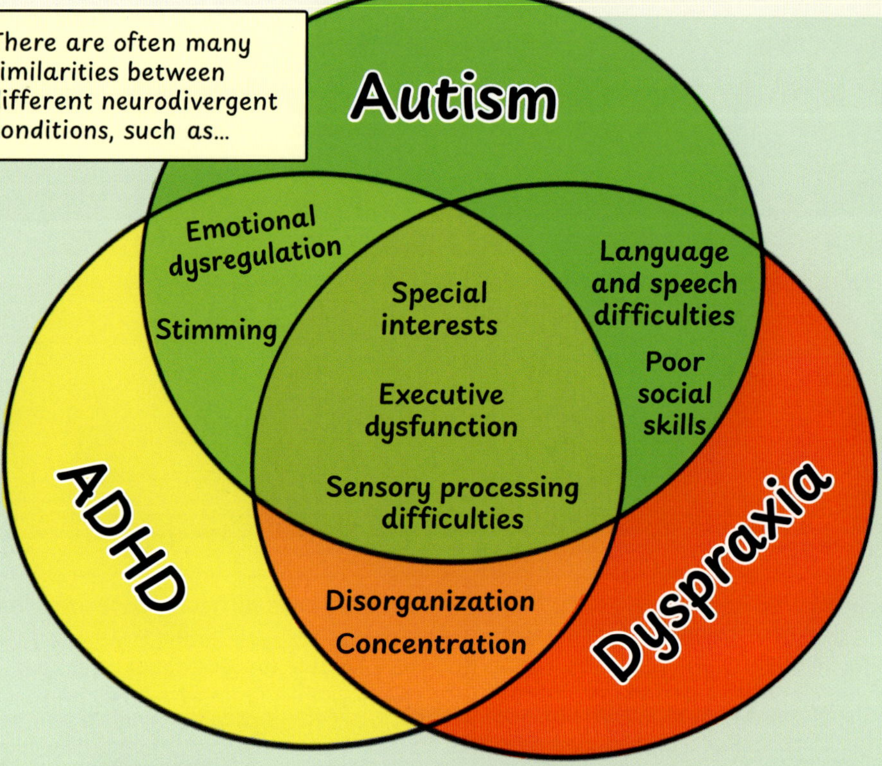

Special interests

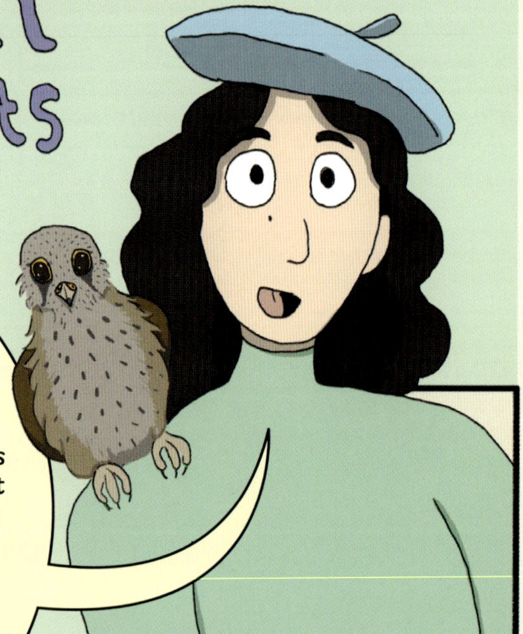

One particular trait that seems to be shared by many different neurodivergent people is having 'special interests'. You may also know of this as 'passions'.

These are interests that we are particularly passionate about. Everyone has interests, but those who are neurodivergent might be more involved with their interests than neurotypicals would be.

You may find yourself obsessed with a particular show, band or period of history. Maybe you watch a lot of documentaries about this subject and read a lot about it to try to learn more. This is how I am with wildlife.

Dyspraxia is sometimes described as an illness, but this is wrong. Dyspraxia is a life-long learning difference that you have from birth and cannot grow out of.

Here is an example of how a dyspraxic person's life might go.

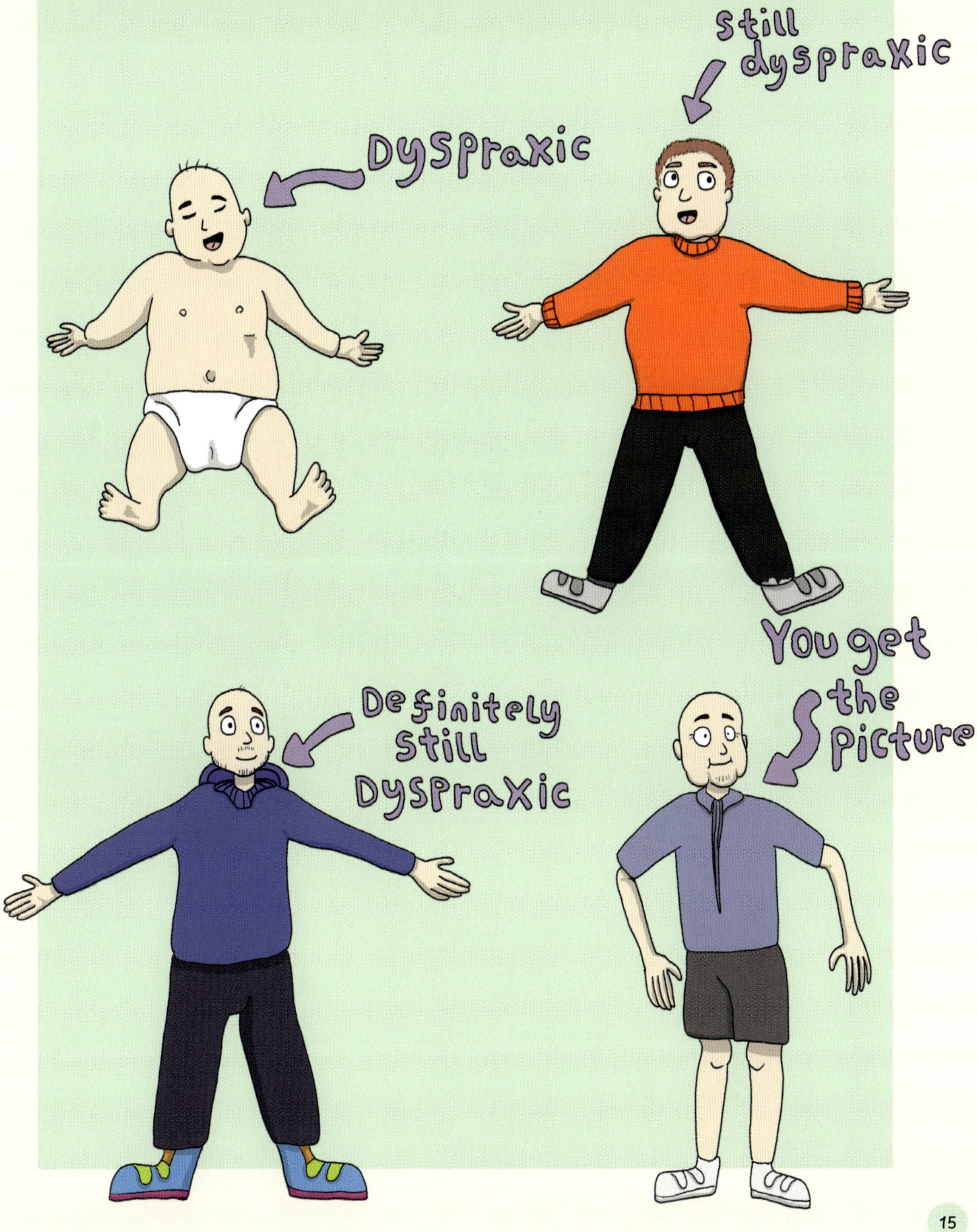

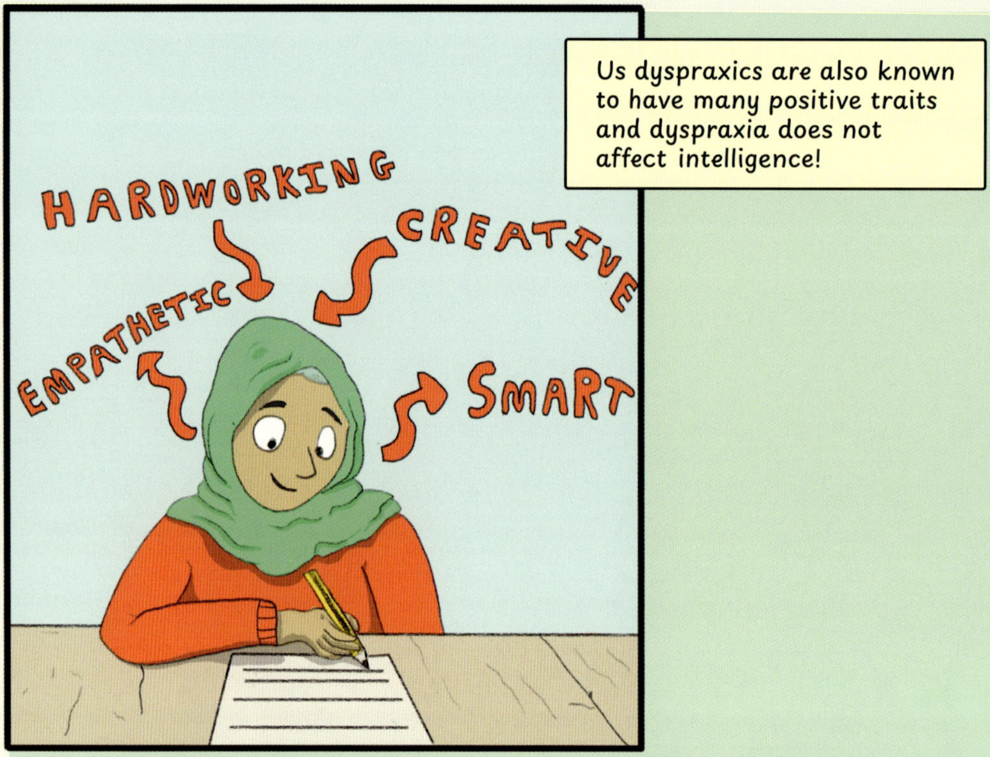
Us dyspraxics are also known to have many positive traits and dyspraxia does not affect intelligence!
HARDWORKING
CREATIVE
EMPATHETIC
SMART

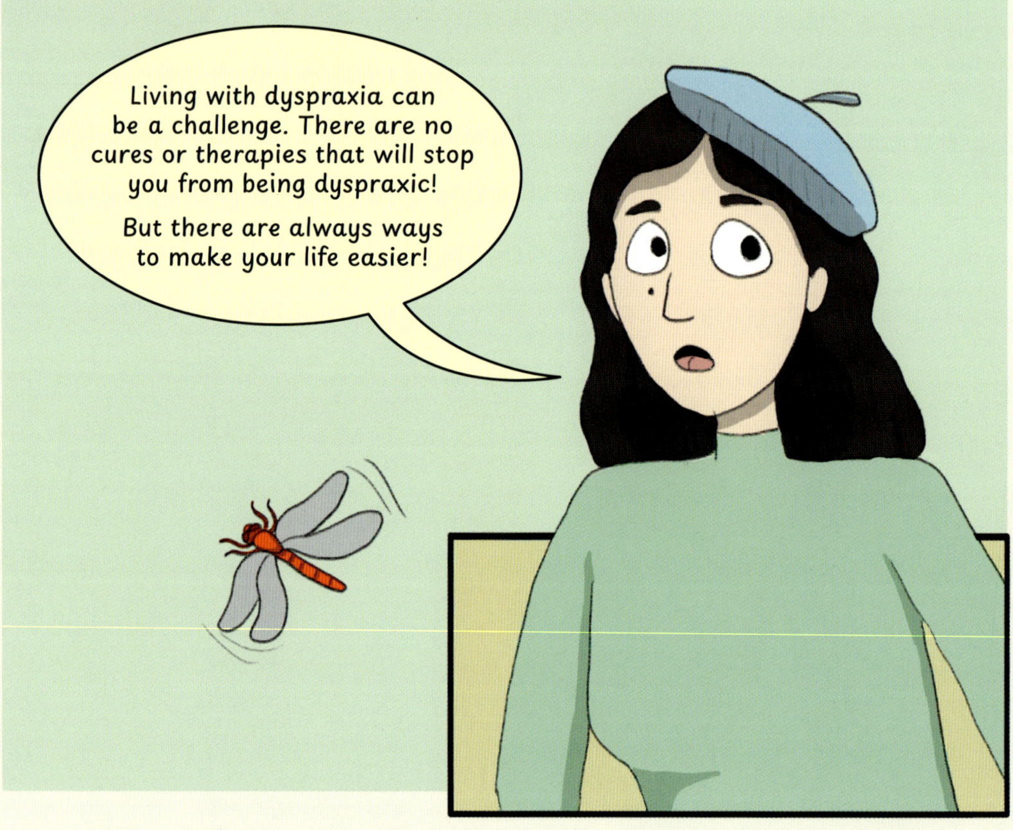
Living with dyspraxia can be a challenge. There are no cures or therapies that will stop you from being dyspraxic!
But there are always ways to make your life easier!

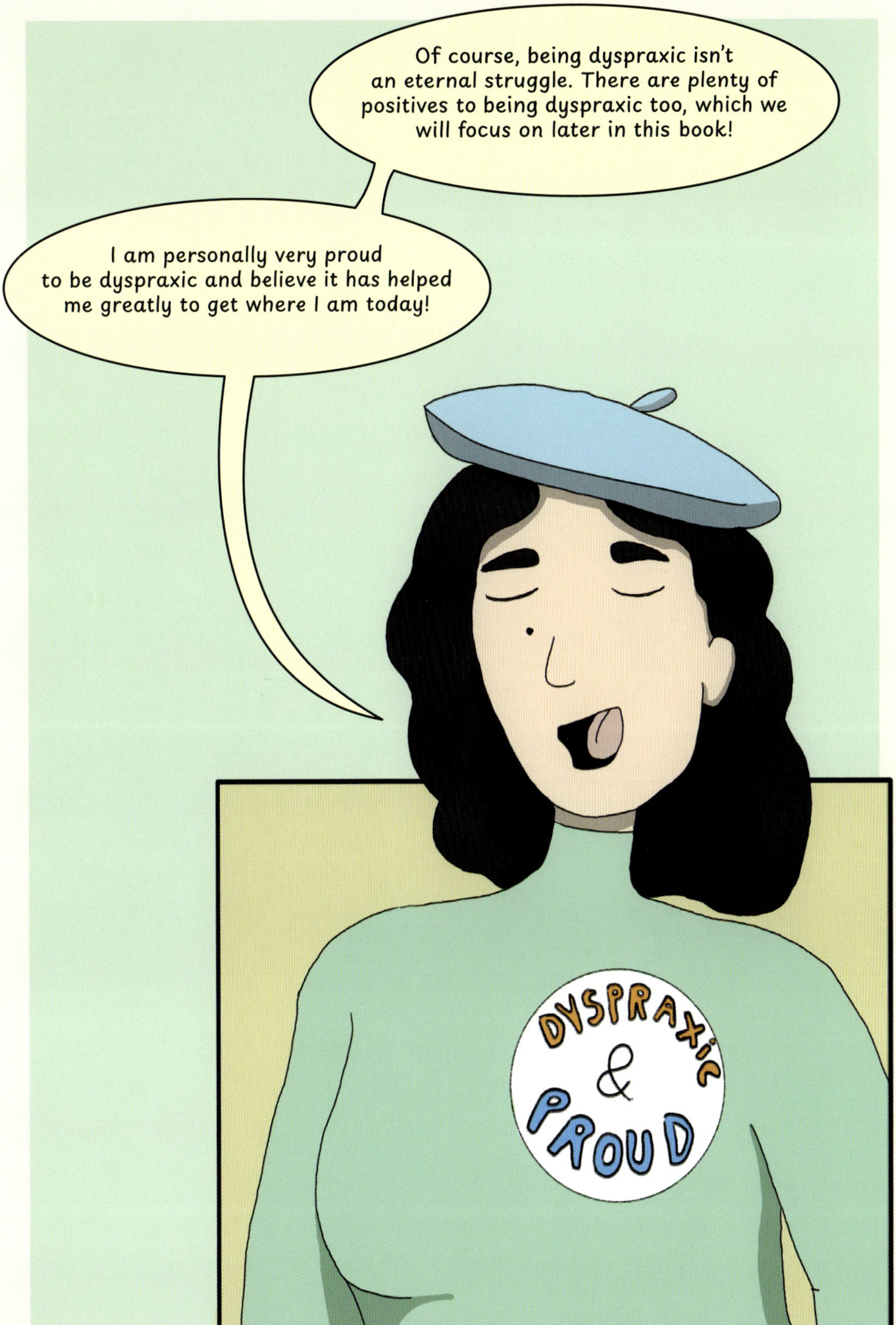
Of course, being dyspraxic isn't an eternal struggle. There are plenty of positives to being dyspraxic too, which we will focus on later in this book!
I am personally very proud to be dyspraxic and believe it has helped me greatly to get where I am today!
DYSPRAXIC & PROUD

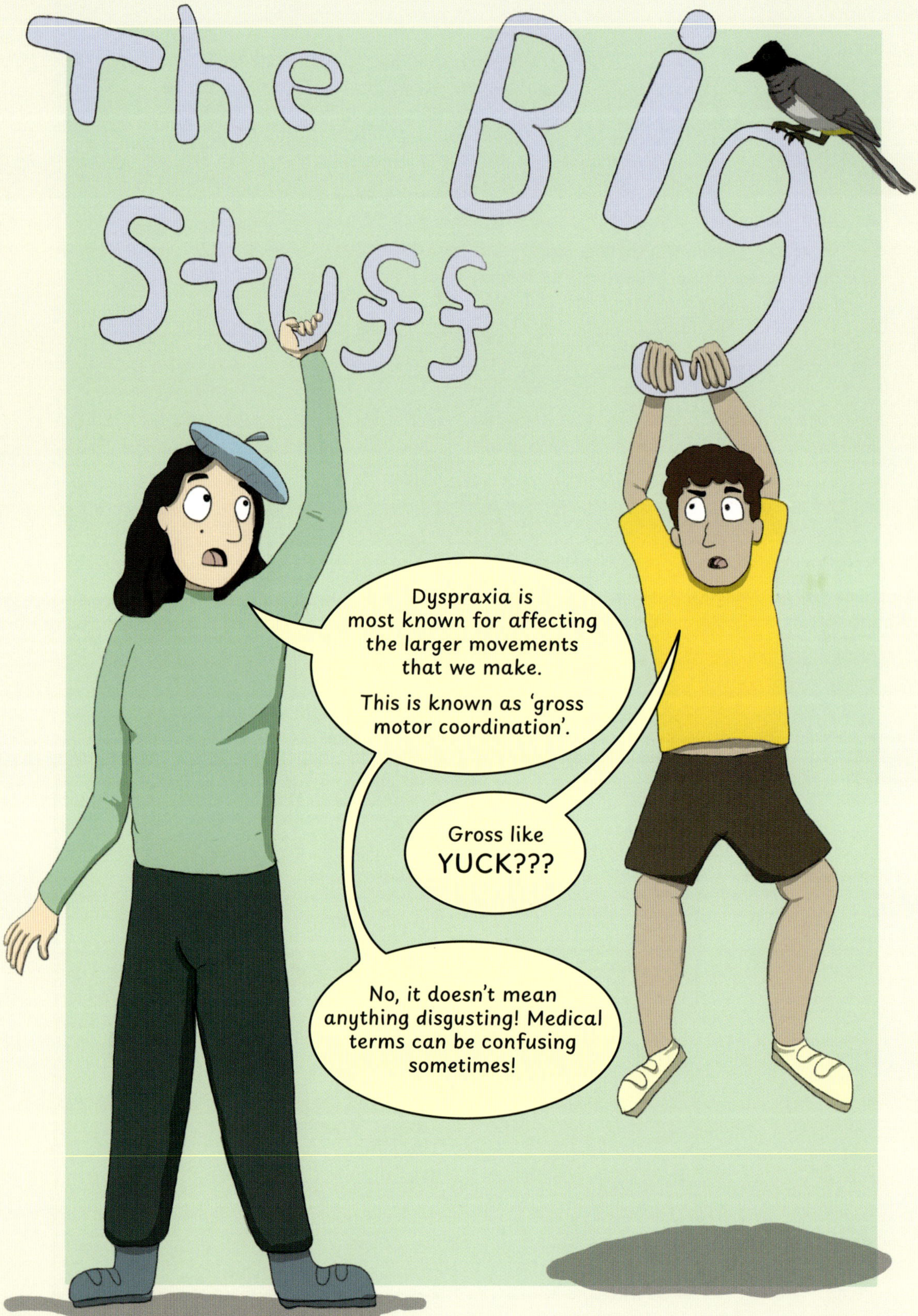
The Big Stuff
Dyspraxia is most known for affecting the larger movements that we make.
This is known as 'gross motor coordination'.
Gross like YUCK???
No, it doesn't mean anything disgusting! Medical terms can be confusing sometimes!

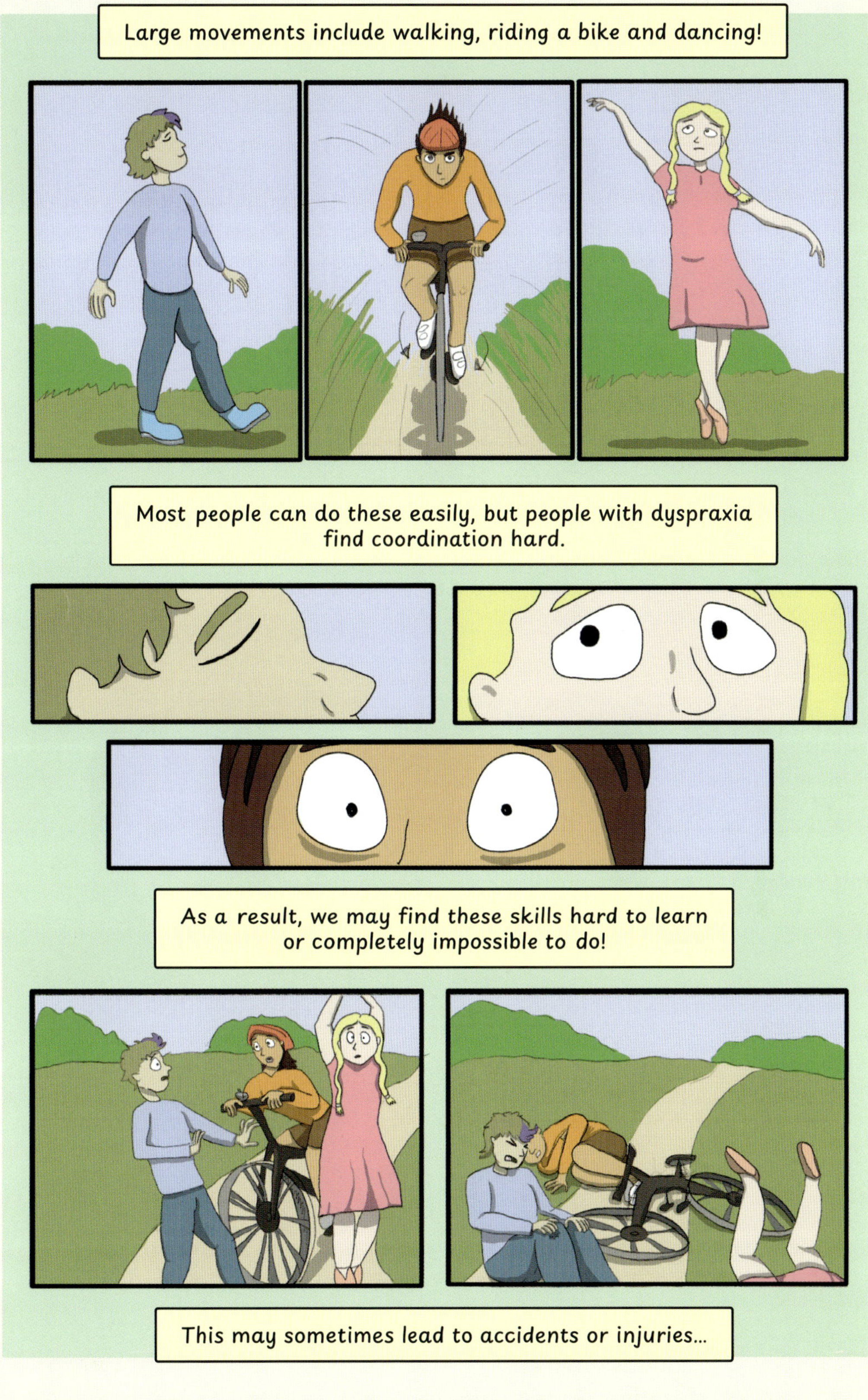
Large movements include walking, riding a bike and dancing!
Most people can do these easily, but people with dyspraxia find coordination hard.
As a result, we may find these skills hard to learn or completely impossible to do!
This may sometimes lead to accidents or injuries...

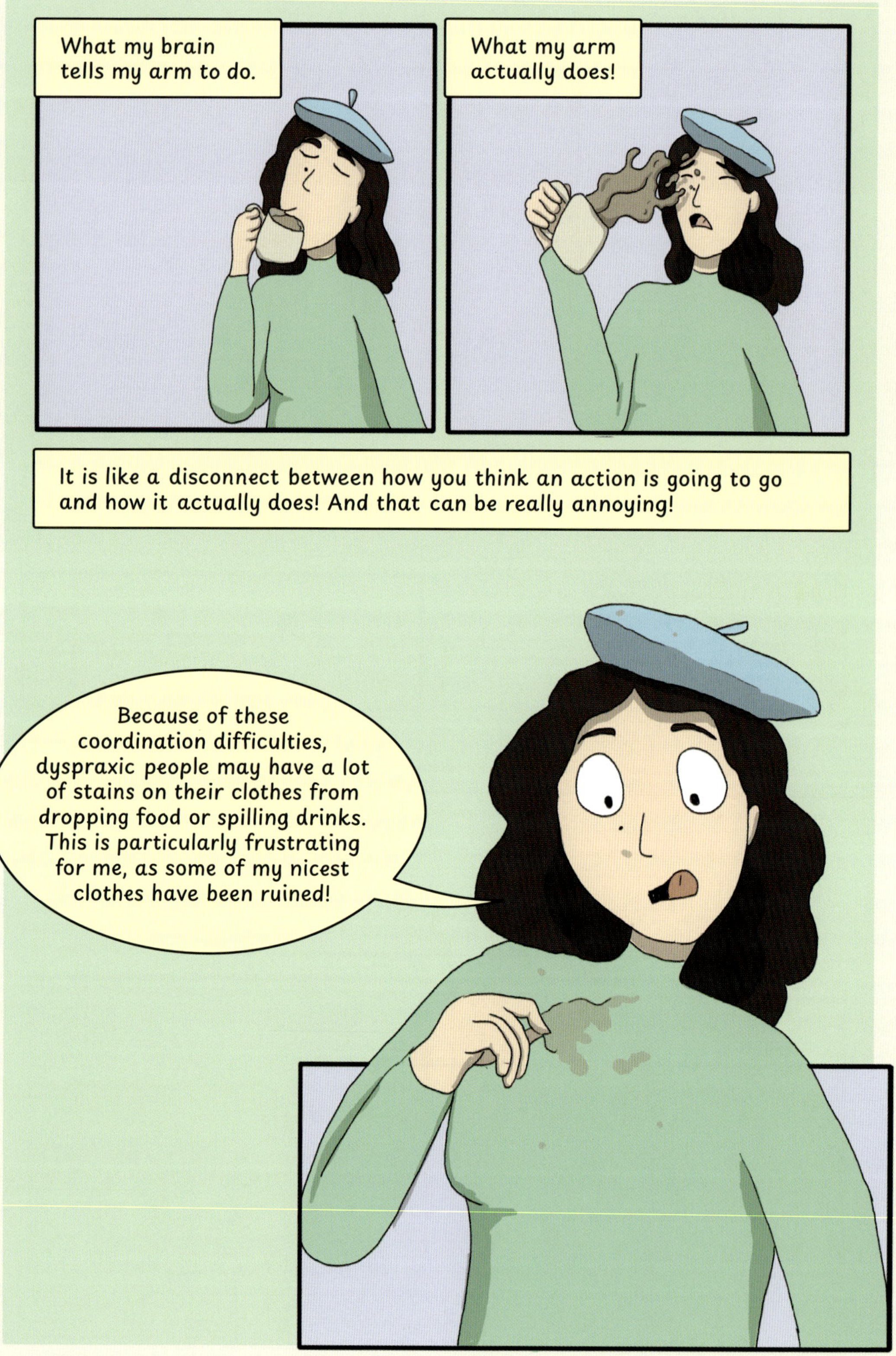
What my brain tells my arm to do.
What my arm actually does!
It is like a disconnect between how you think an action is going to go and how it actually does! And that can be really annoying!
Because of these coordination difficulties, dyspraxic people may have a lot of stains on their clothes from dropping food or spilling drinks. This is particularly frustrating for me, as some of my nicest clothes have been ruined!

The lack of gross motor coordination is most known for affecting dyspraxics' ability to play sports. This can mean that we struggle in lessons like PE, but there are other ways that dyspraxia can impact our everyday lives.

Here is what a bad day could look like!

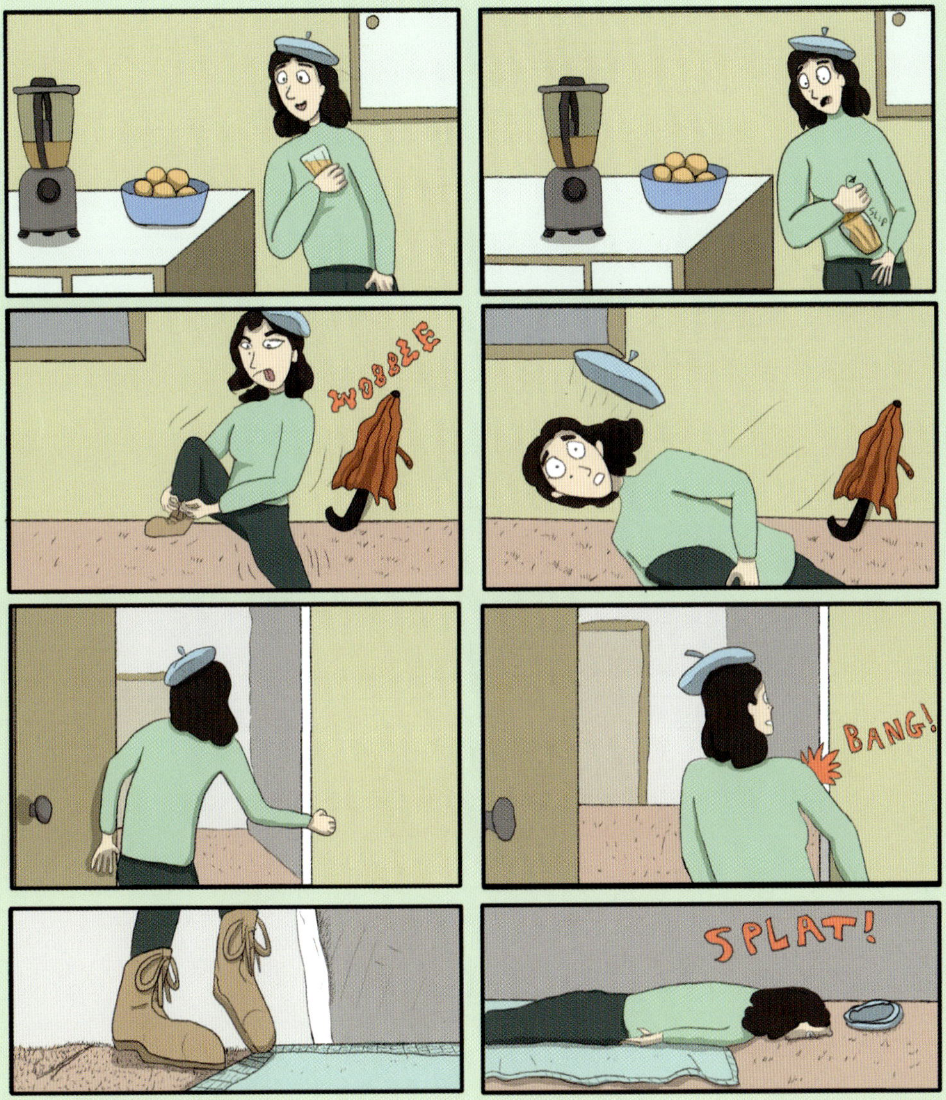

How our dyspraxia impacts us can change from day to day. Some days I may find myself to be more clumsy than others. A lot of it depends on how tired I am, which means that getting enough sleep is very important to me!

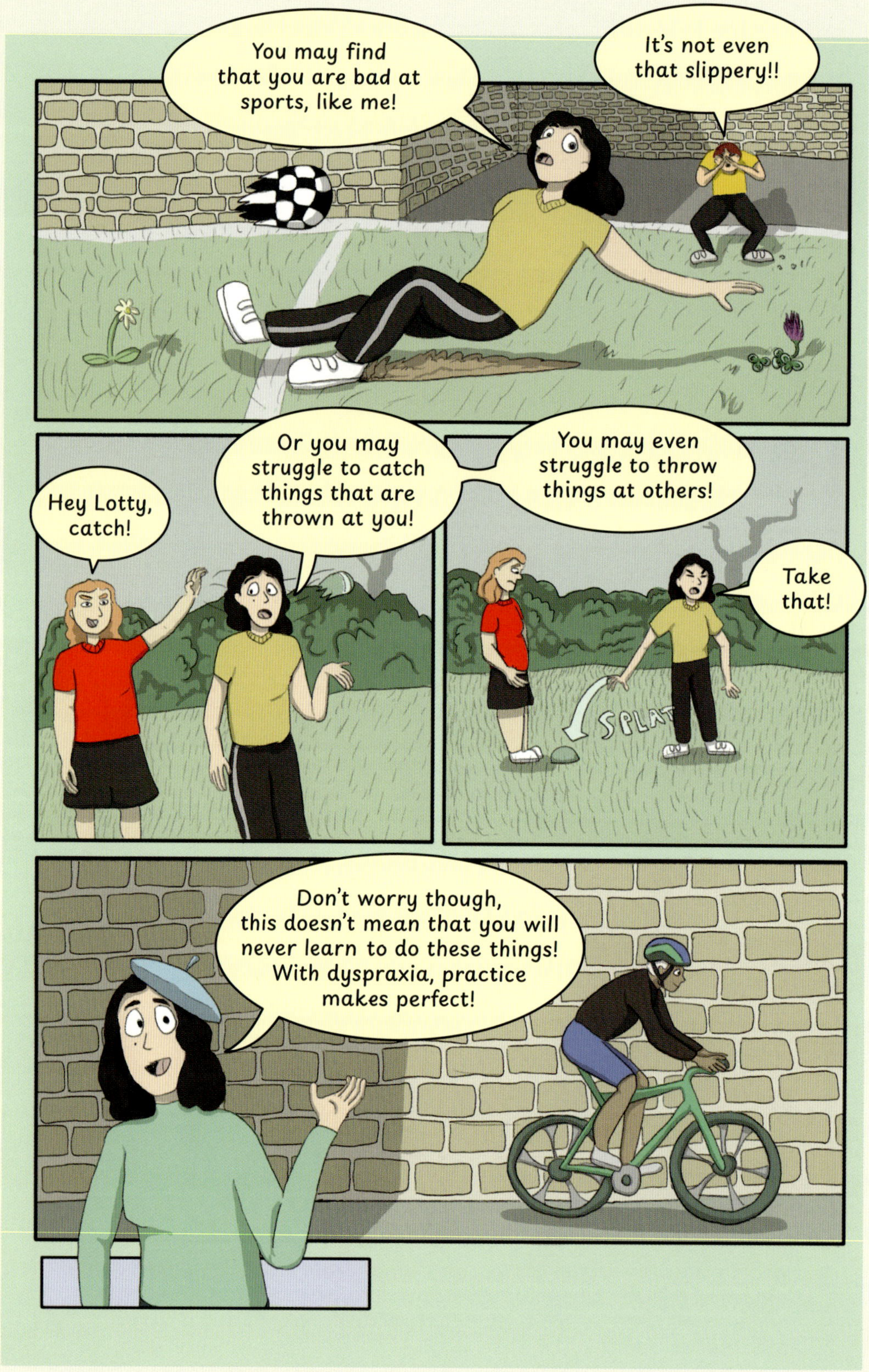
You may find that you are bad at sports, like me!
It's not even that slippery!!
Hey Lotty, catch!
Or you may struggle to catch things that are thrown at you!
You may even struggle to throw things at others!
Take that!
SPLAT
Don't worry though, this doesn't mean that you will never learn to do these things! With dyspraxia, practice makes perfect!

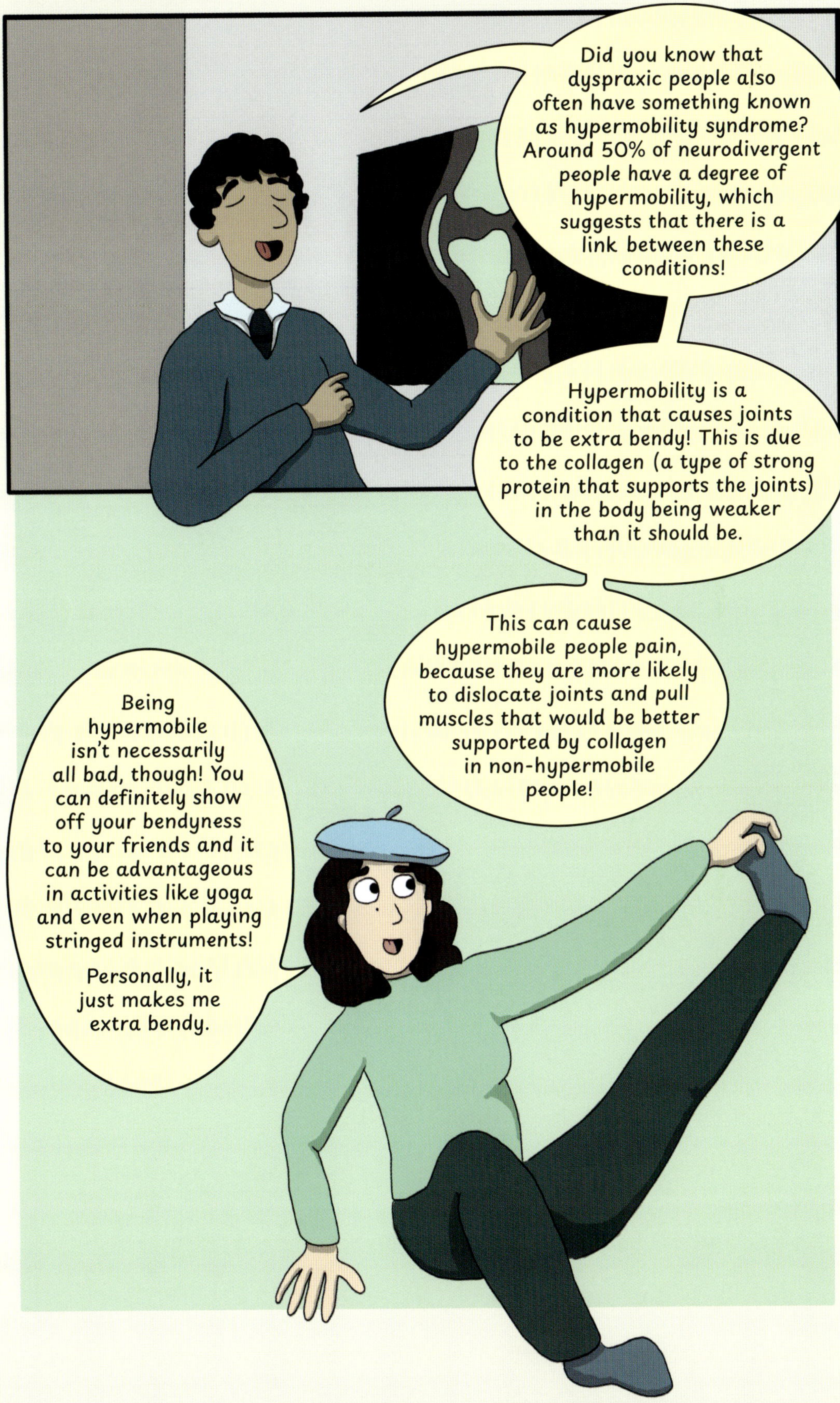
Did you know that dyspraxic people also often have something known as hypermobility syndrome? Around 50% of neurodivergent people have a degree of hypermobility, which suggests that there is a link between these conditions!
Hypermobility is a condition that causes joints to be extra bendy! This is due to the collagen (a type of strong protein that supports the joints) in the body being weaker than it should be.
This can cause hypermobile people pain, because they are more likely to dislocate joints and pull muscles that would be better supported by collagen in non-hypermobile people!
Being hypermobile isn't necessarily all bad, though! You can definitely show off your bendyness to your friends and it can be advantageous in activities like yoga and even when playing stringed instruments!
Personally, it just makes me extra bendy.

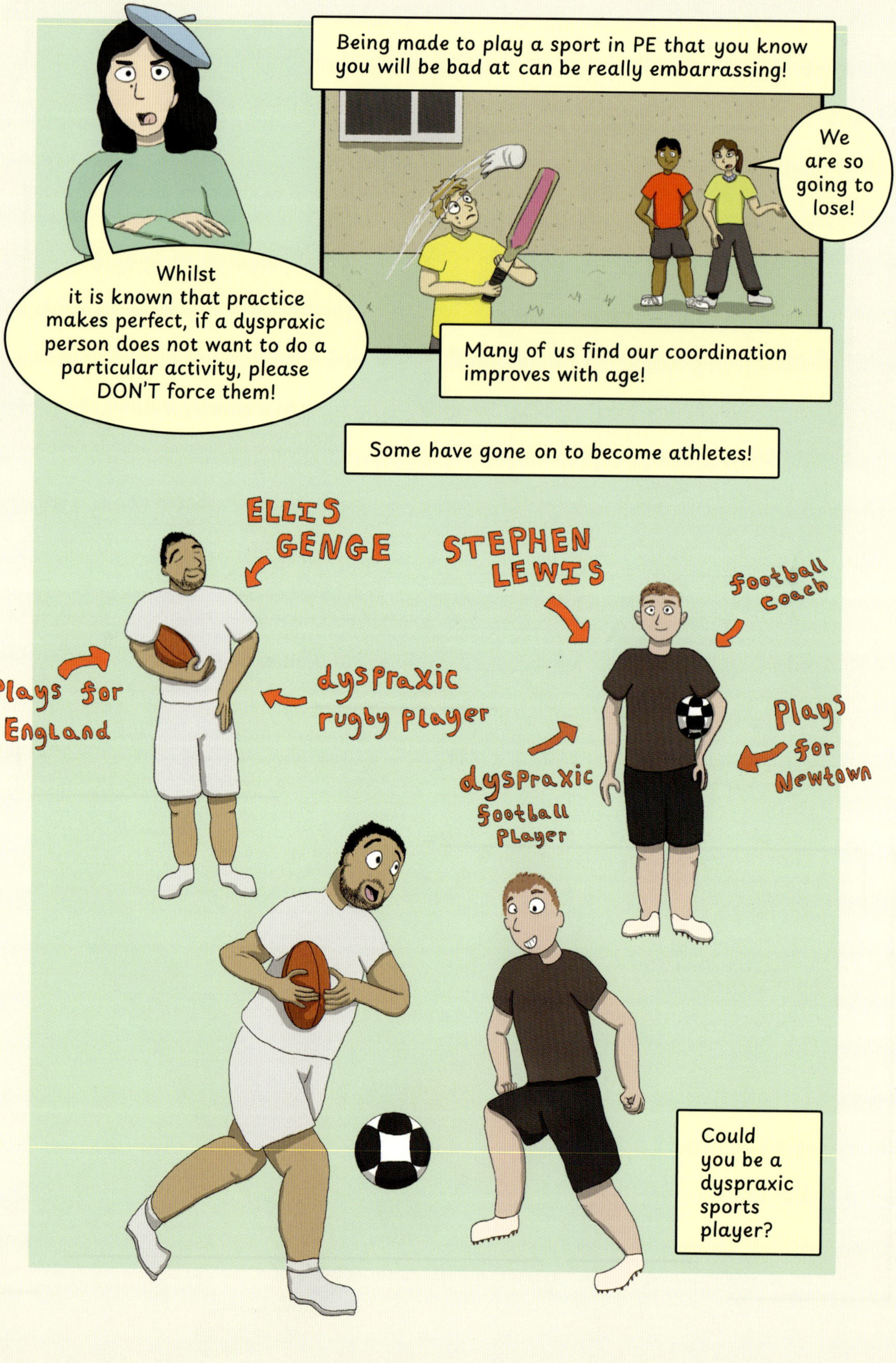
Being made to play a sport in PE that you know you will be bad at can be really embarrassing!
We are so going to lose!
Whilst it is known that practice makes perfect, if a dyspraxic person does not want to do a particular activity, please DON'T force them!
Many of us find our coordination improves with age!
Some have gone on to become athletes!
ELLIS GENGE
Plays for England
dyspraxic rugby player
STEPHEN LEWIS
football coach
Plays for Newtown
dyspraxic football player
Could you be a dyspraxic sports player?

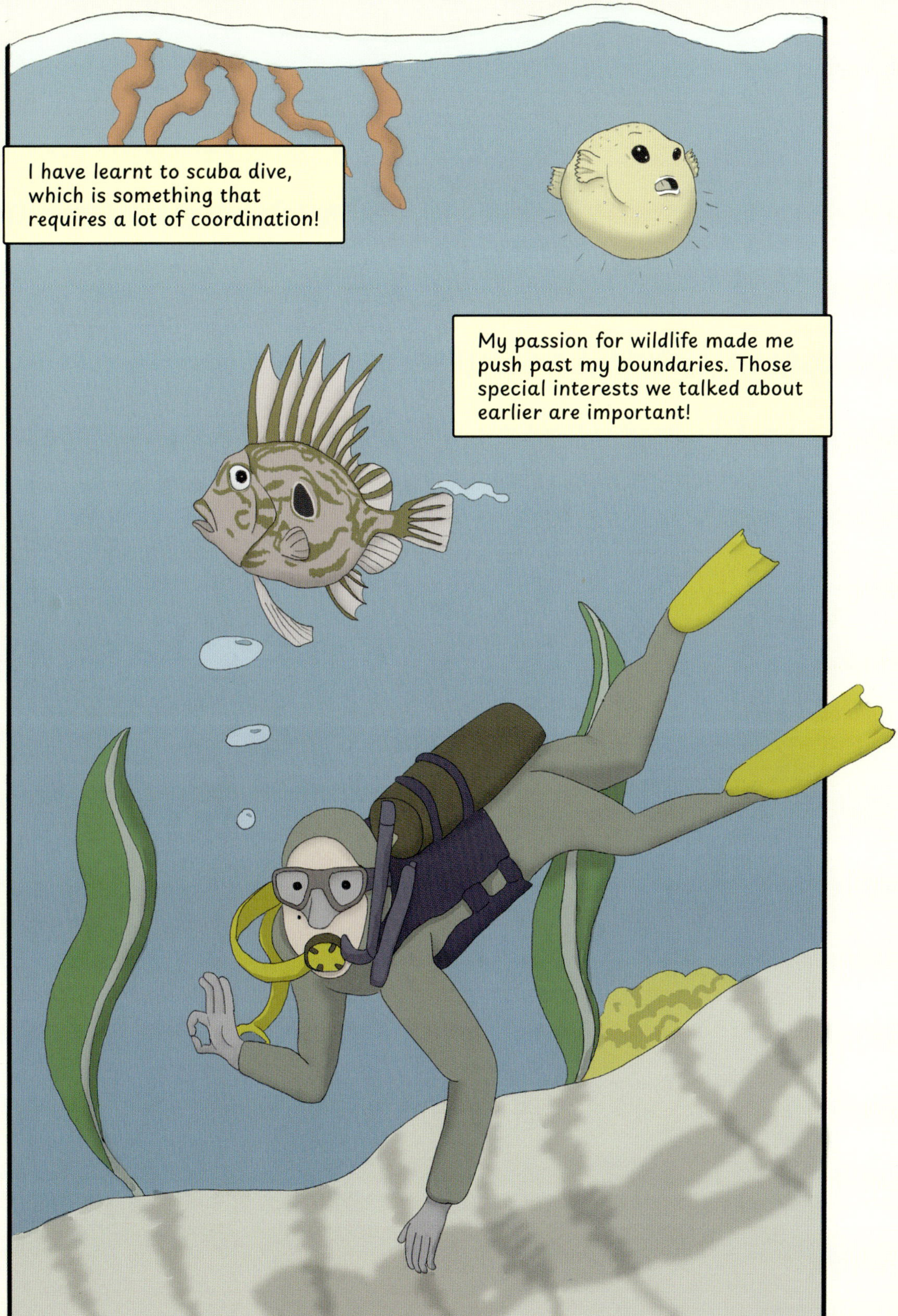
I have learnt to scuba dive, which is something that requires a lot of coordination!
My passion for wildlife made me push past my boundaries. Those special interests we talked about earlier are important!

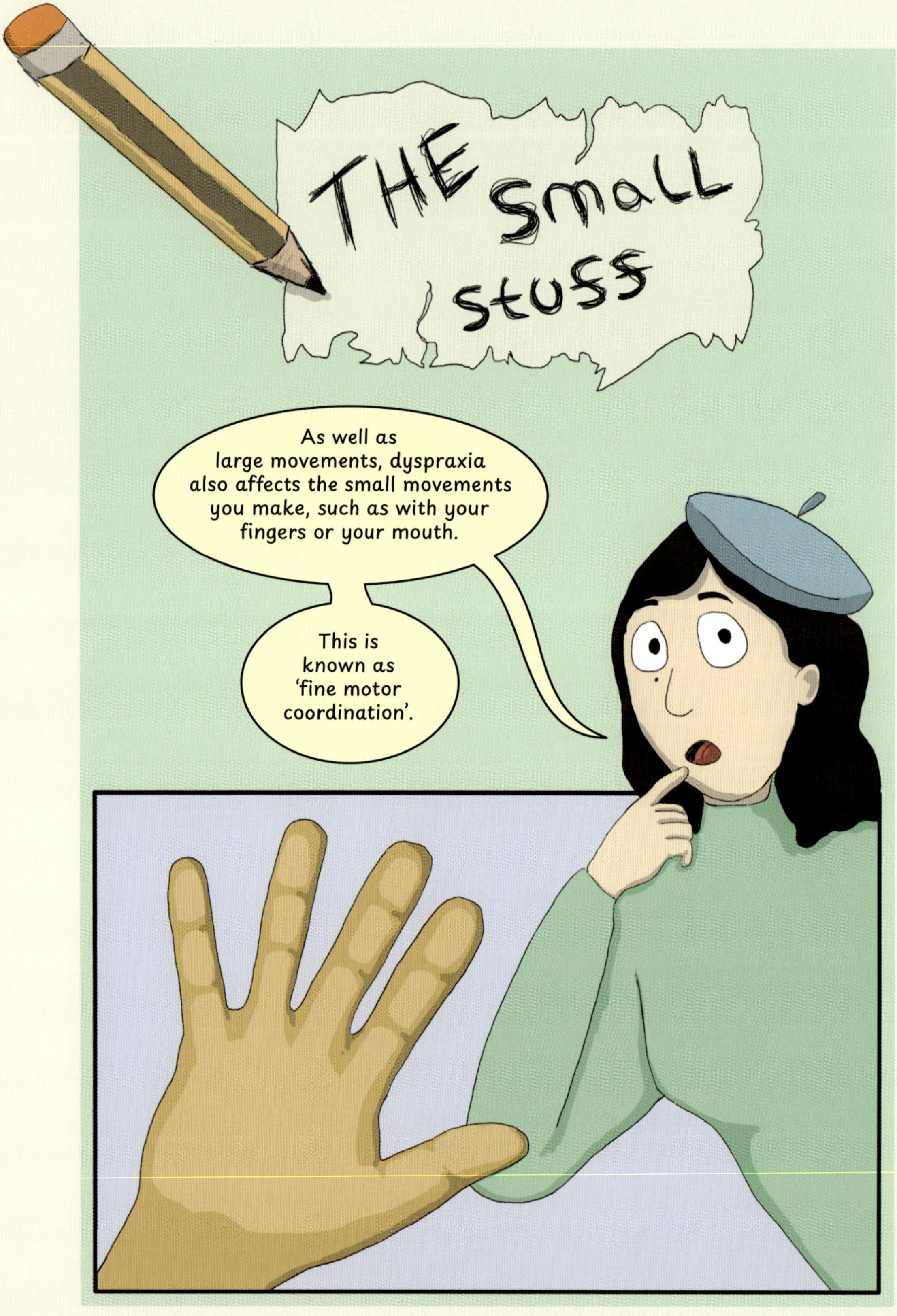
THE Small stuff
As well as large movements, dyspraxia also affects the small movements you make, such as with your fingers or your mouth.
This is known as 'fine motor coordination'.

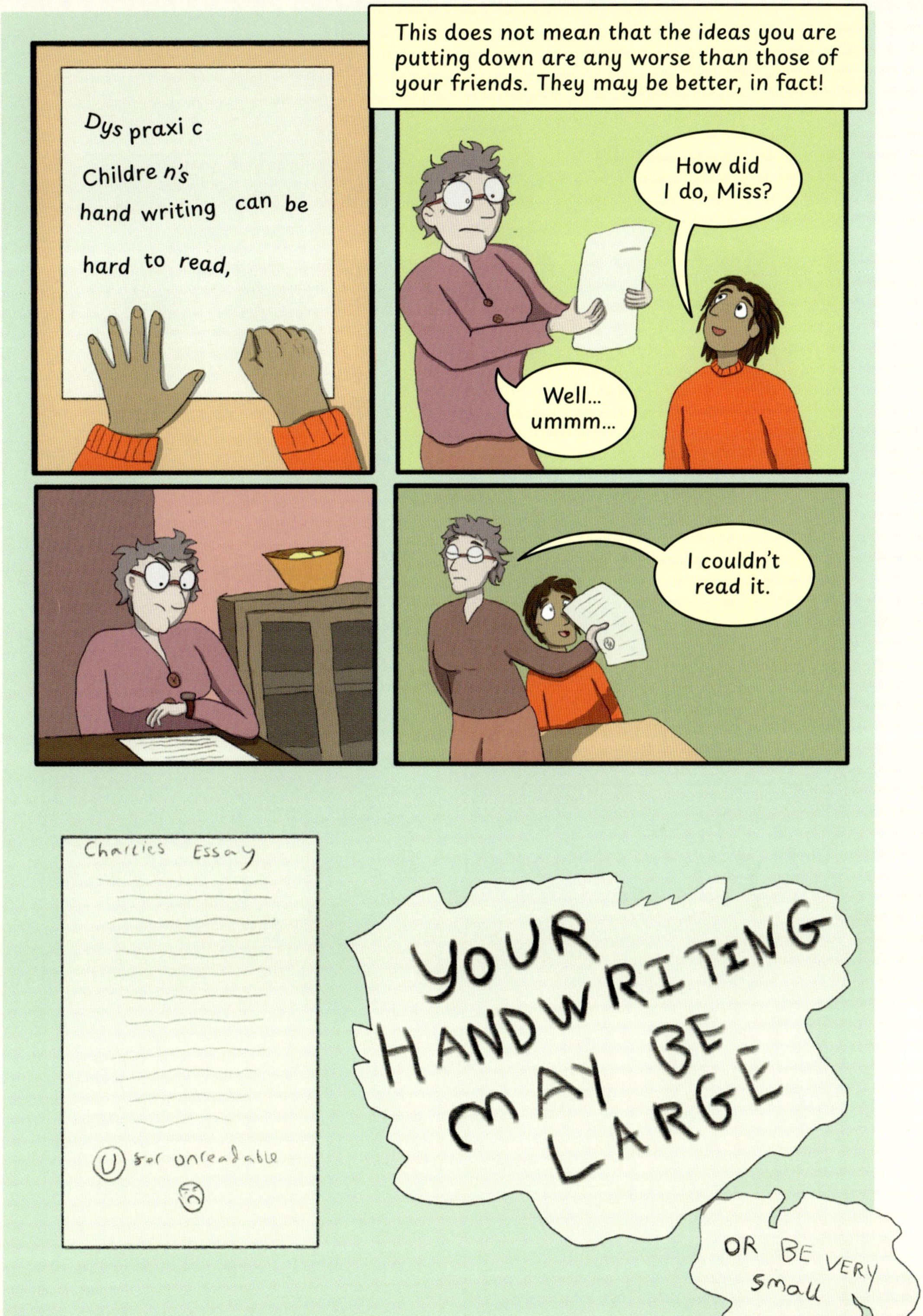
This does not mean that the ideas you are putting down are any worse than those of your friends. They may be better, in fact!
Dys praxi c Childre n's hand writing can be hard to read,
How did I do, Miss?
Well... ummm...
I couldn't read it.
Charlies Essay
U for unreadable
YOUR HANDWRITING MAY BE LARGE
OR BE VERY small

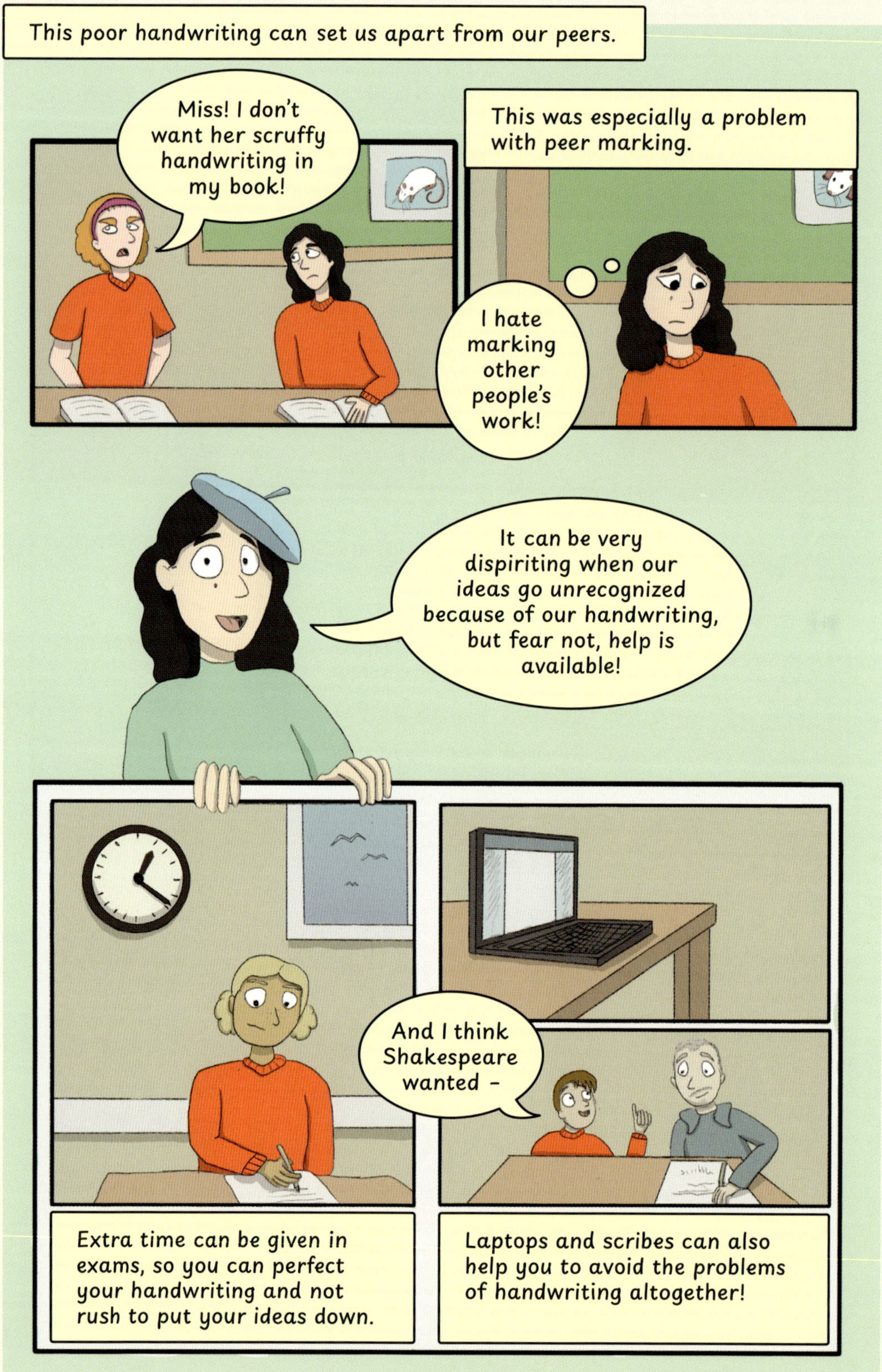
This poor handwriting can set us apart from our peers.
Miss! I don't want her scruffy handwriting in my book!
This was especially a problem with peer marking.
I hate marking other people's work!
It can be very dispiriting when our ideas go unrecognized because of our handwriting, but fear not, help is available!
And I think Shakespeare wanted –
Extra time can be given in exams, so you can perfect your handwriting and not rush to put your ideas down.
Laptops and scribes can also help you to avoid the problems of handwriting altogether!

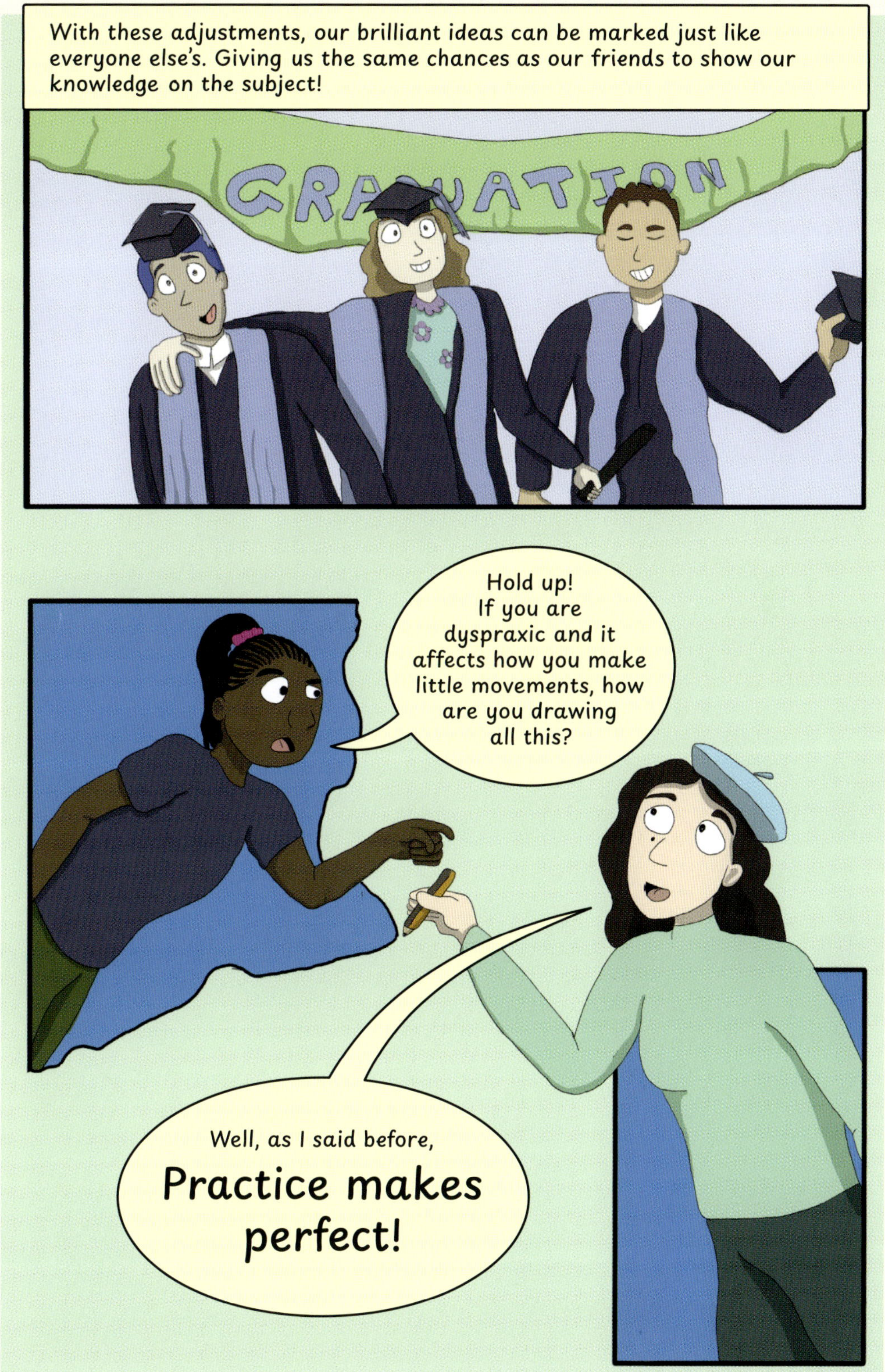
With these adjustments, our brilliant ideas can be marked just like everyone else's. Giving us the same chances as our friends to show our knowledge on the subject!
GRADUATION
Hold up! If you are dyspraxic and it affects how you make little movements, how are you drawing all this?
Well, as I said before, Practice makes perfect!

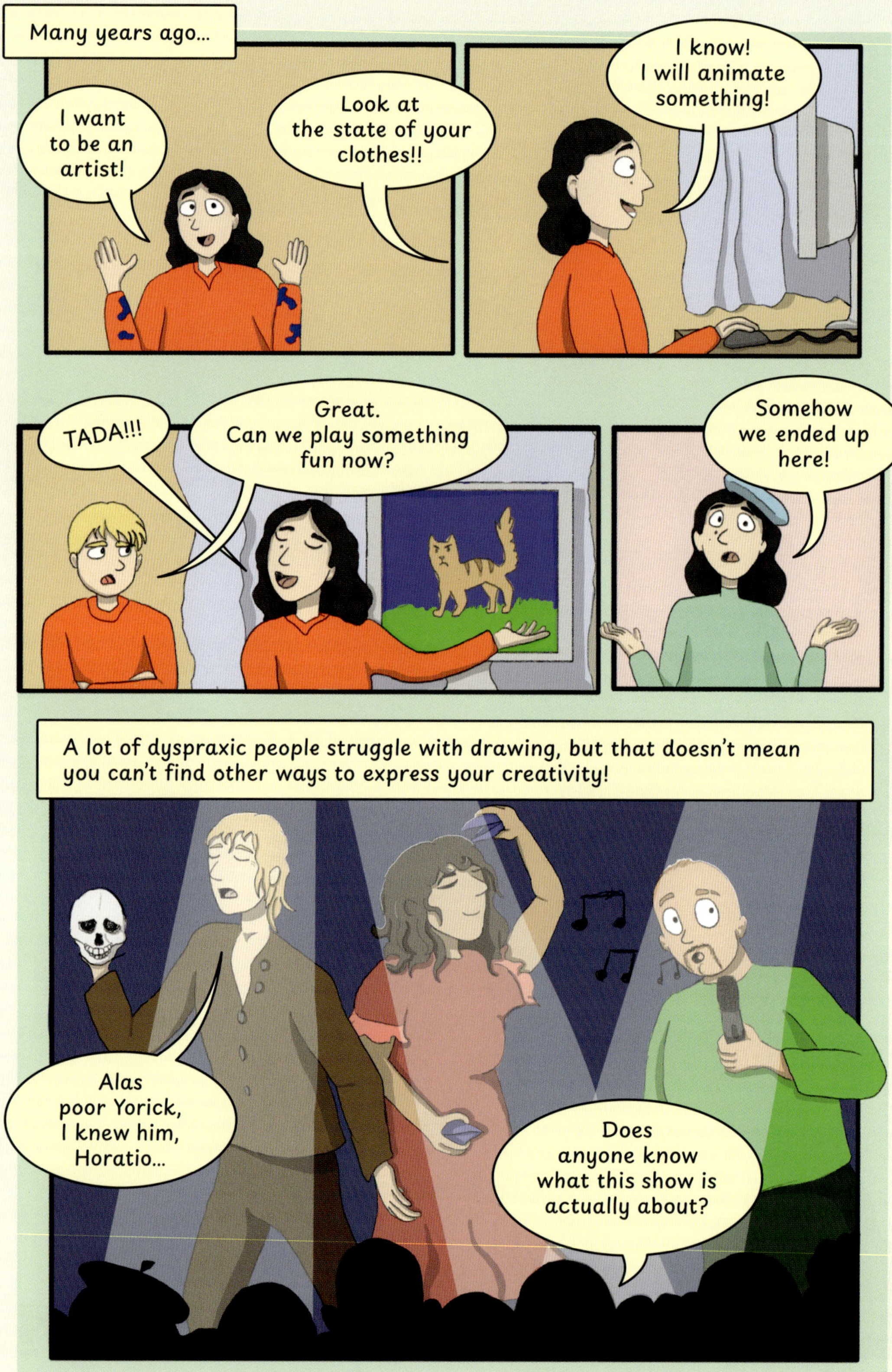
Many years ago...
I want to be an artist!
Look at the state of your clothes!!
I know! I will animate something!
TADA!!!
Great. Can we play something fun now?
Somehow we ended up here!
A lot of dyspraxic people struggle with drawing, but that doesn't mean you can't find other ways to express your creativity!
Alas poor Yorick, I knew him, Horatio...
Does anyone know what this show is actually about?

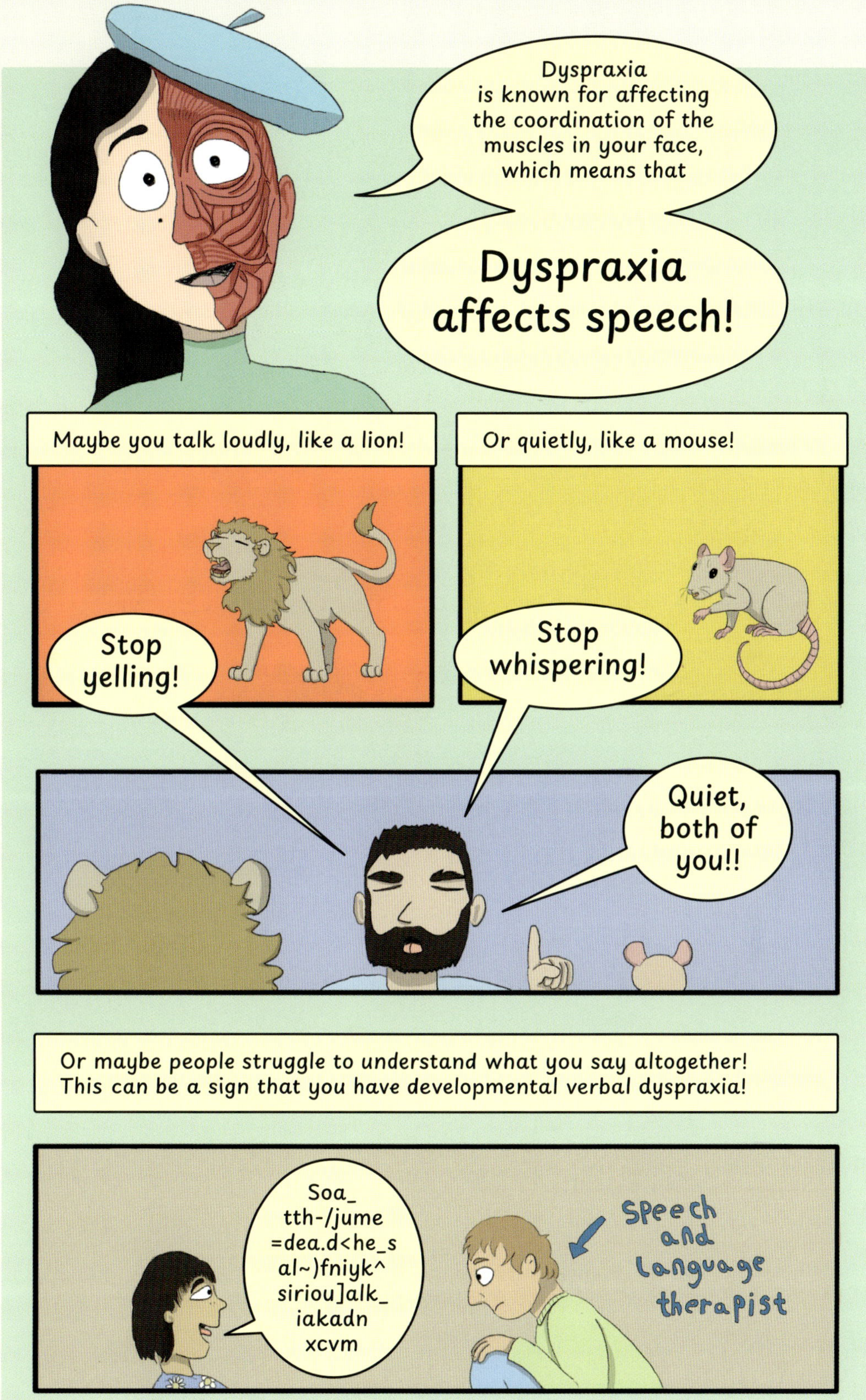

Dyspraxia is known for affecting the coordination of the muscles in your face, which means that
Dyspraxia affects speech!
Maybe you talk loudly, like a lion!
Or quietly, like a mouse!
Stop yelling!
Stop whispering!
Quiet, both of you!!
Or maybe people struggle to understand what you say altogether! This can be a sign that you have developmental verbal dyspraxia!
Soa_ tth-/jume =dea.d<he_s al~)fniyk^ siriou]alk_ iakadn xcvm
Speech and Language therapist

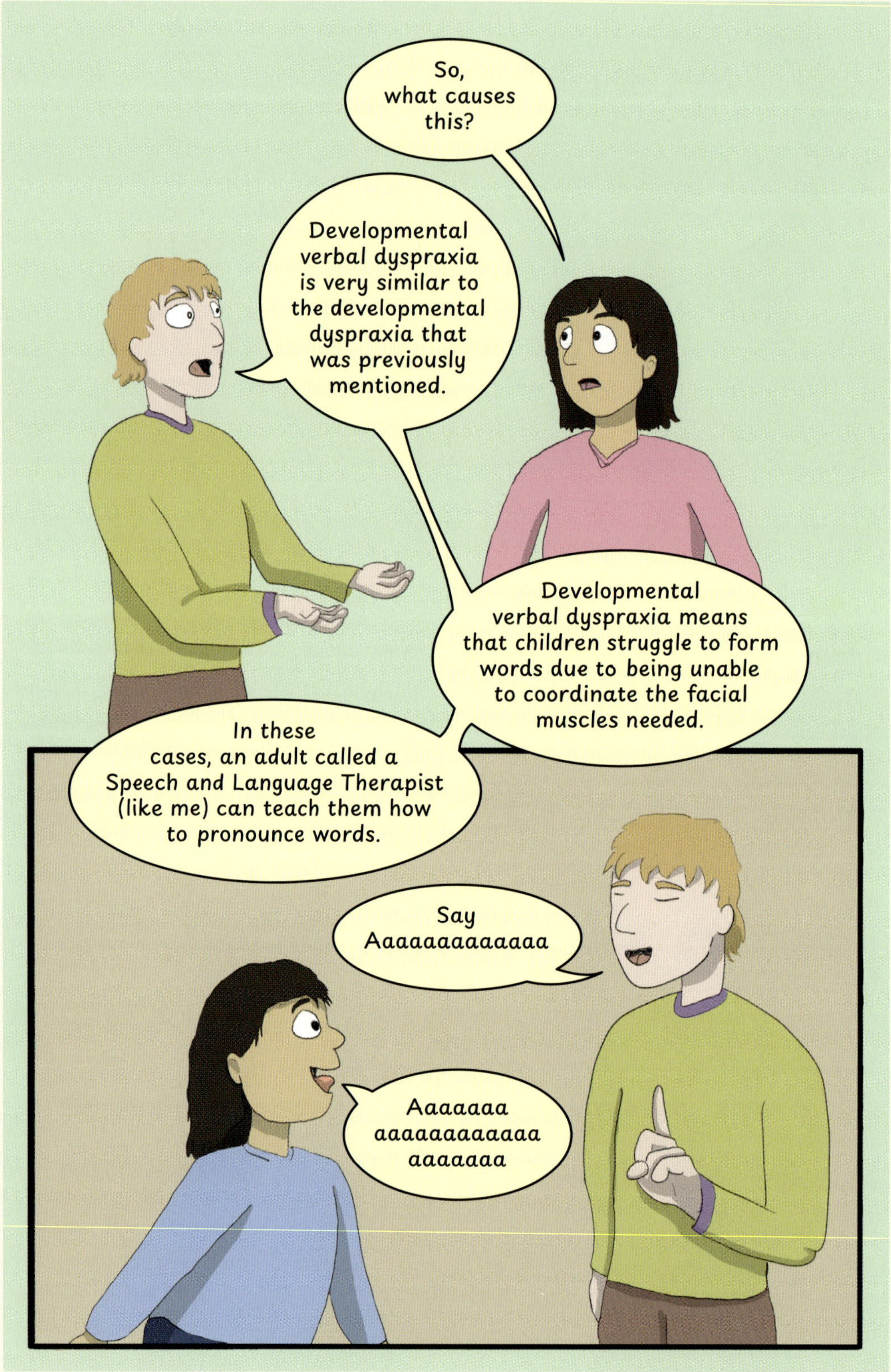
So, what causes this?
Developmental verbal dyspraxia is very similar to the developmental dyspraxia that was previously mentioned.
Developmental verbal dyspraxia means that children struggle to form words due to being unable to coordinate the facial muscles needed.
In these cases, an adult called a Speech and Language Therapist (like me) can teach them how to pronounce words.
Say Aaaaaaaaaaaa
Aaaaaaa aaaaaaaaaaa aaaaaaa

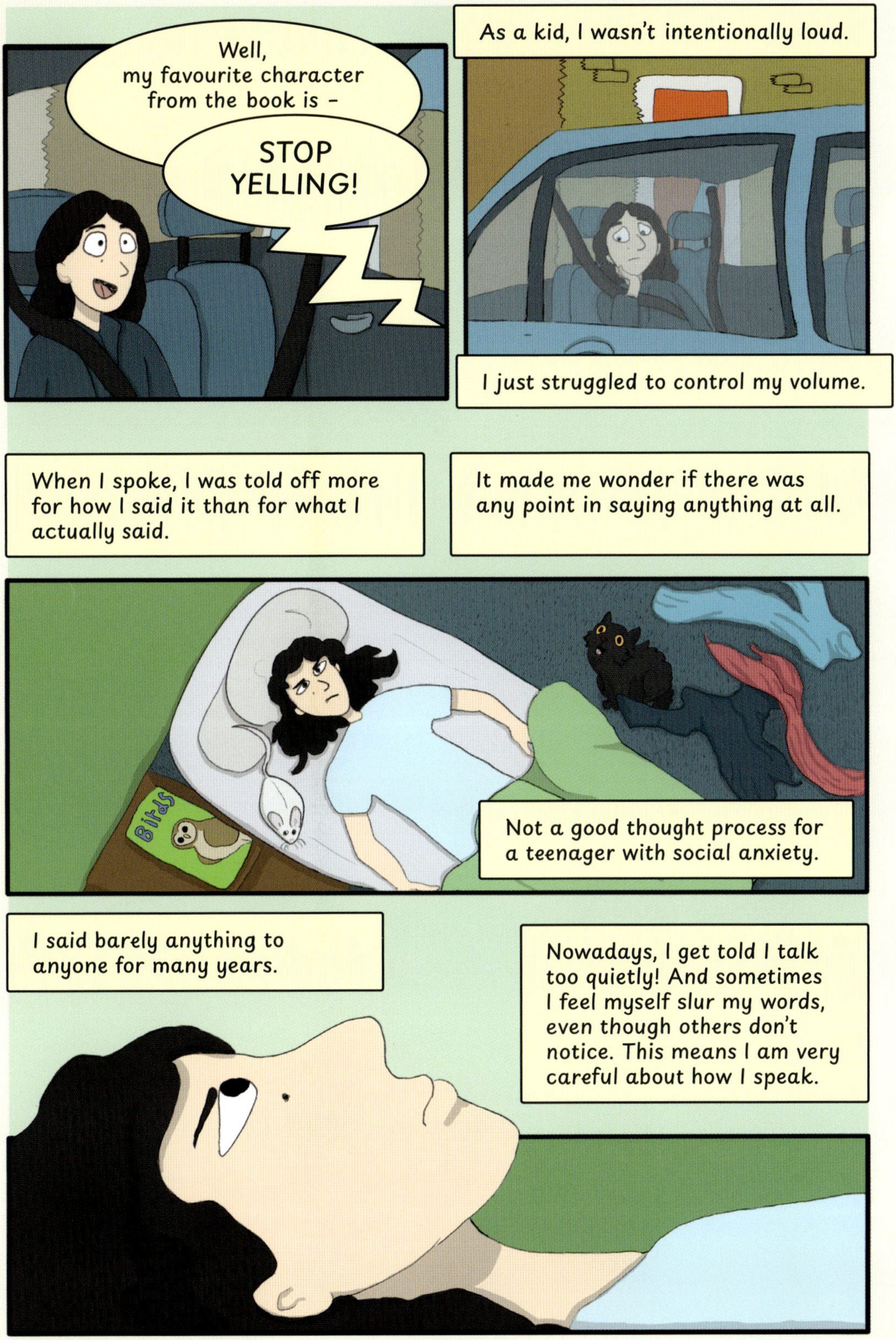

Well, my favourite character from the book is –
STOP YELLING!
As a kid, I wasn't intentionally loud.
I just struggled to control my volume.
When I spoke, I was told off more for how I said it than for what I actually said.
It made me wonder if there was any point in saying anything at all.
Birds
Not a good thought process for a teenager with social anxiety.
I said barely anything to anyone for many years.
Nowadays, I get told I talk too quietly! And sometimes I feel myself slur my words, even though others don't notice. This means I am very careful about how I speak.

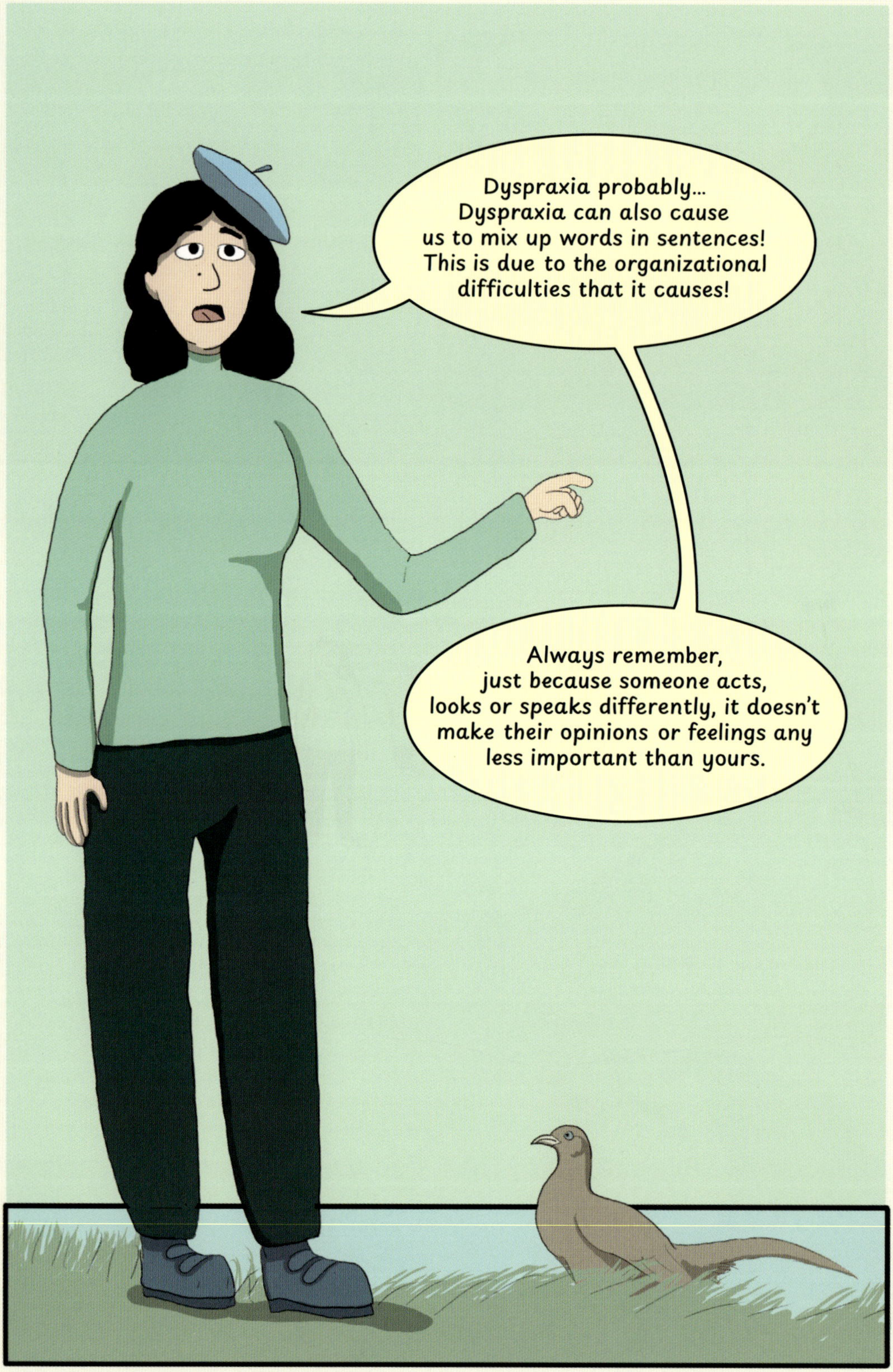
Dyspraxia probably... Dyspraxia can also cause us to mix up words in sentences! This is due to the organizational difficulties that it causes!
Always remember, just because someone acts, looks or speaks differently, it doesn't make their opinions or feelings any less important than yours.

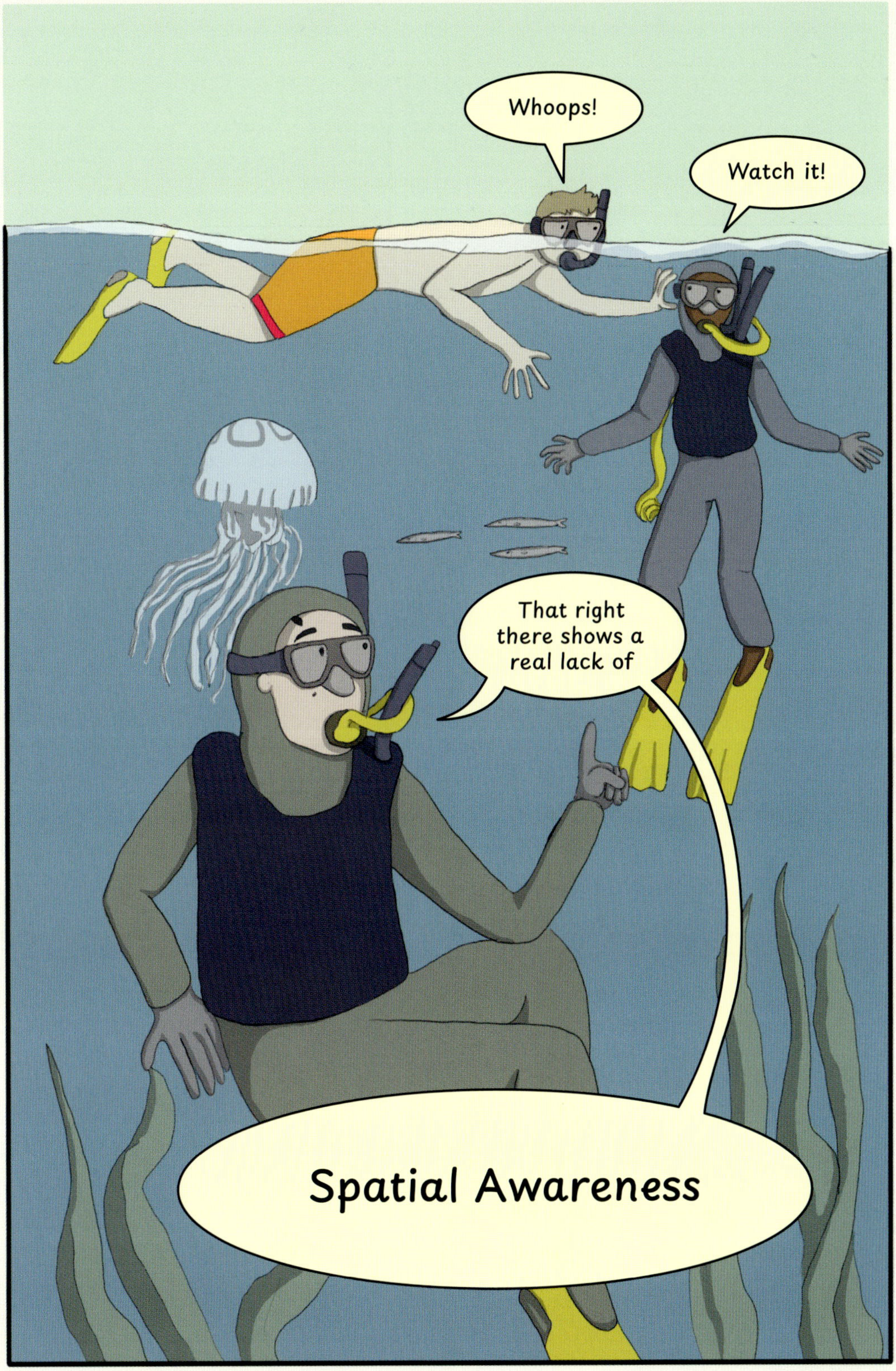
Whoops!
Watch it!
That right there shows a real lack of
Spatial Awareness

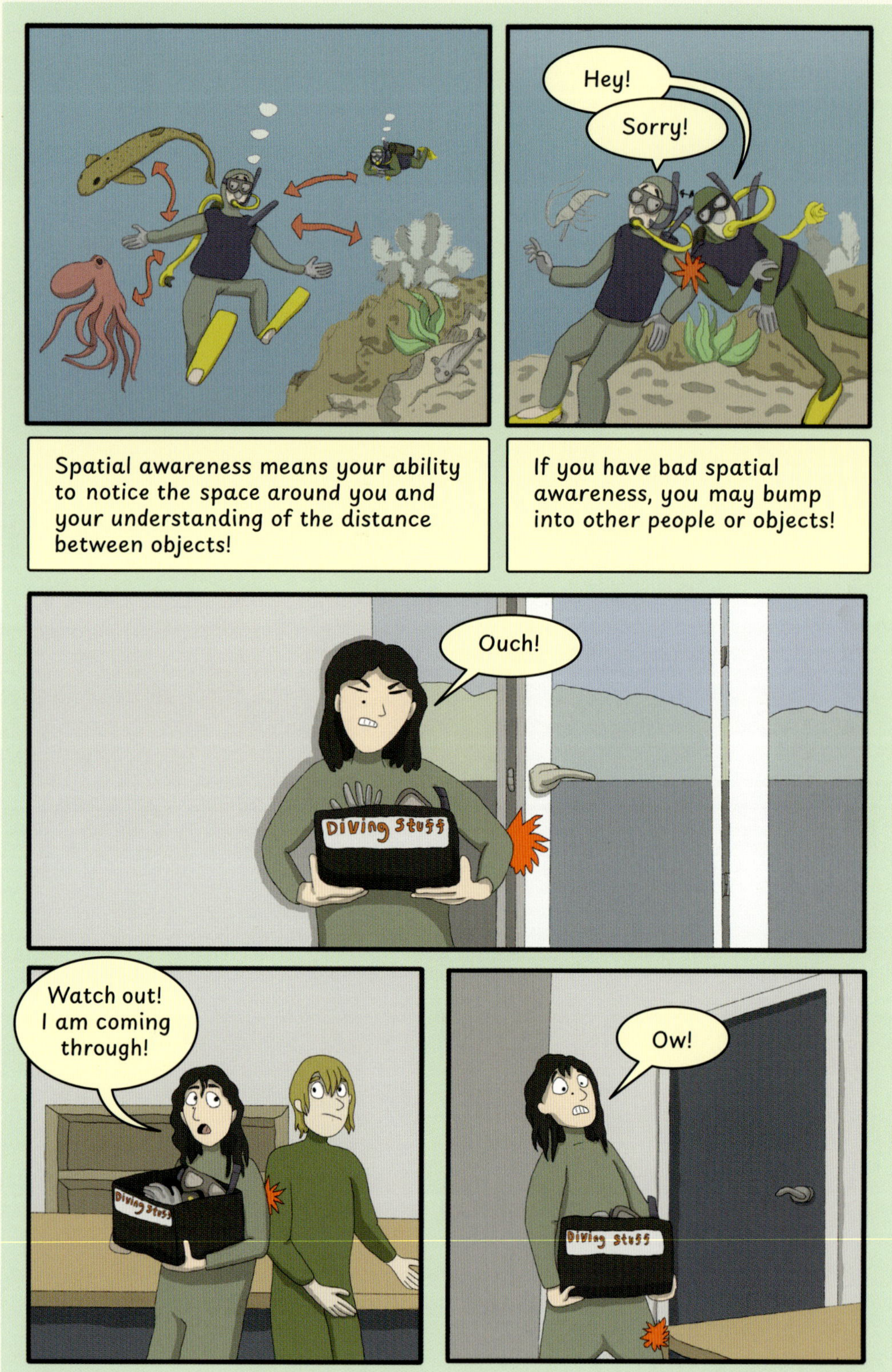
Hey!
Sorry!
Spatial awareness means your ability to notice the space around you and your understanding of the distance between objects!
If you have bad spatial awareness, you may bump into other people or objects!
Ouch!
Diving Stuff
Watch out! I am coming through!
Diving Stuff
Ow!
Diving Stuff

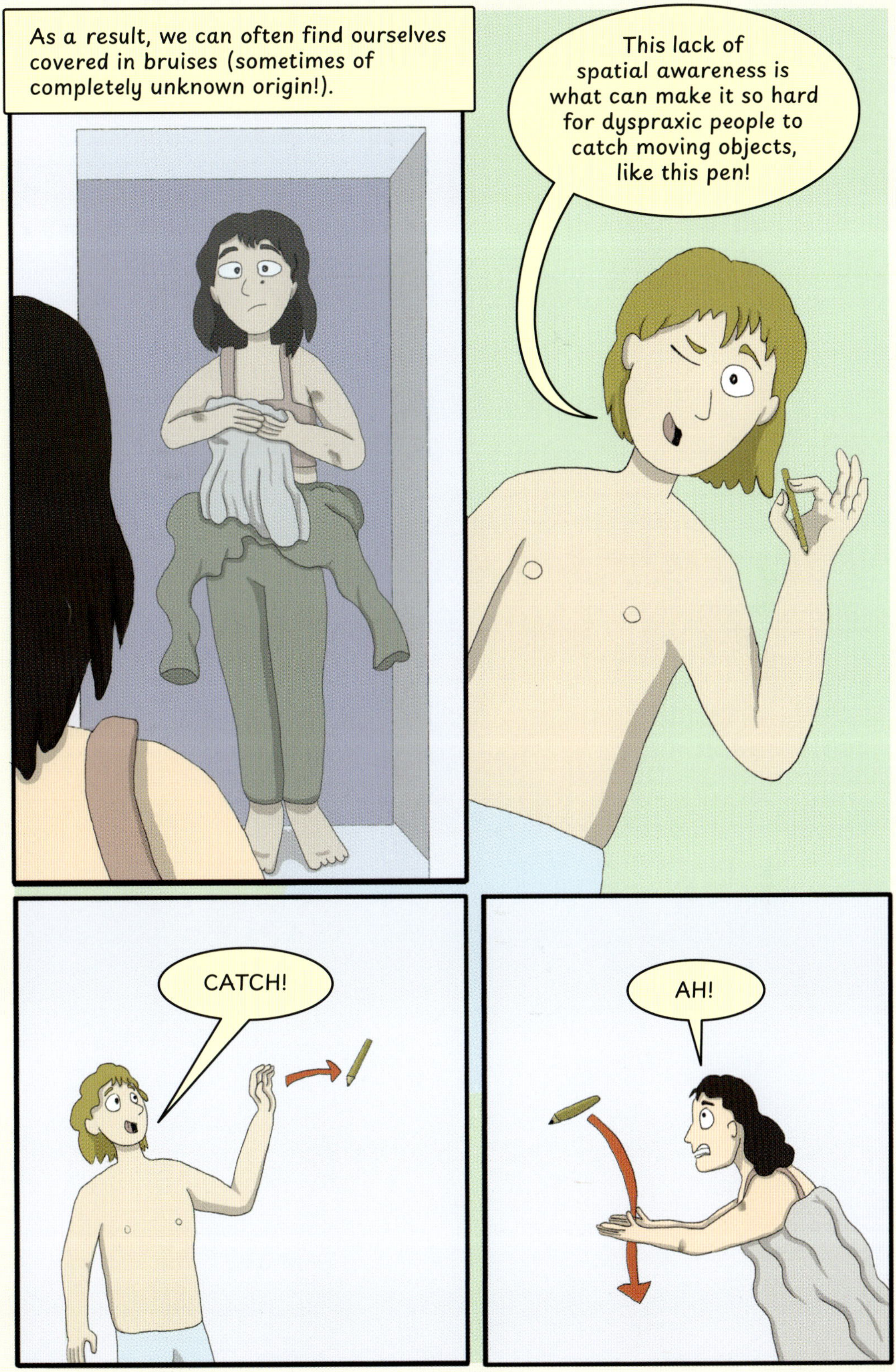
As a result, we can often find ourselves covered in bruises (sometimes of completely unknown origin!).
This lack of spatial awareness is what can make it so hard for dyspraxic people to catch moving objects, like this pen!
CATCH!
AH!

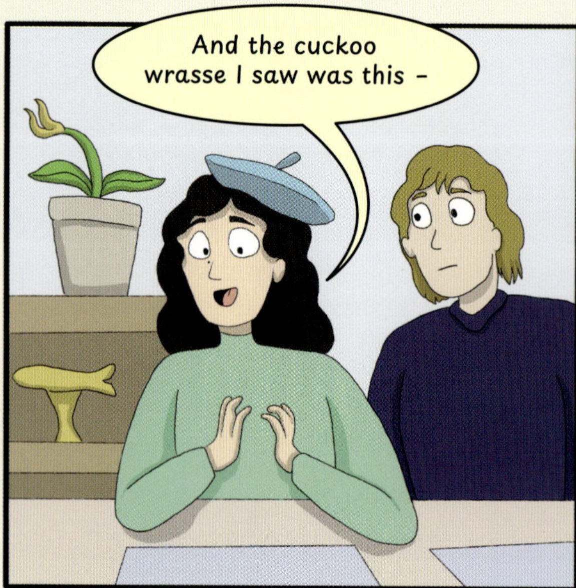

Spatial awareness can also impact our sense of where the smaller parts of our body are and how fast they are moving!

We don't have good control over how small or large our movements are either, so an attempt at a small hand movement might lead to a slap in the face for whichever unfortunate person is standing too close.

This is something some of my friends have experienced, especially when I am talking about something I am passionate about (I tend to wave my hands around a lot!).

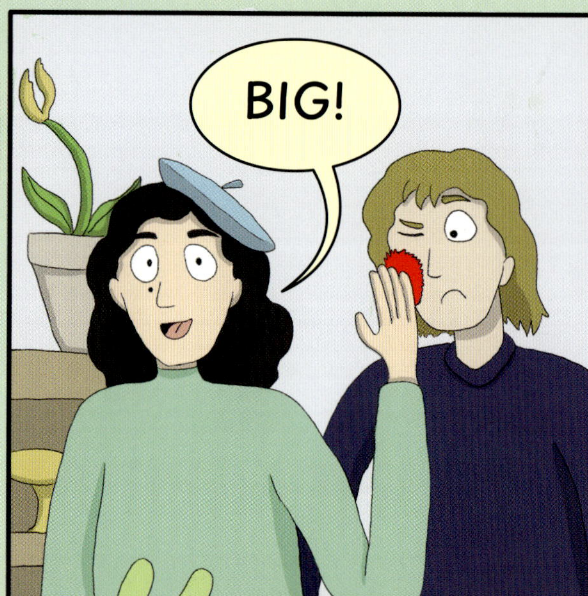

Dyspraxic people often struggle to tell the difference between left and right.

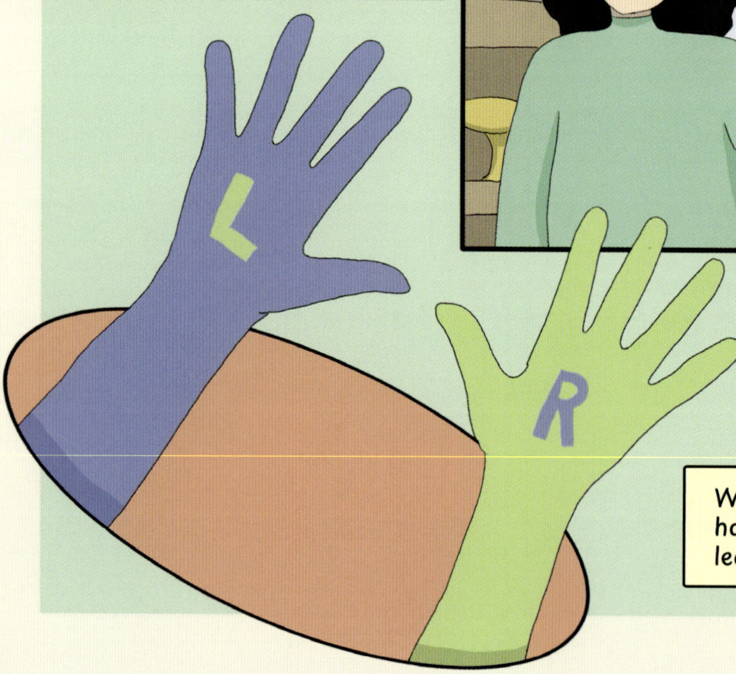

Writing L and R on your hands can help you to learn the difference!

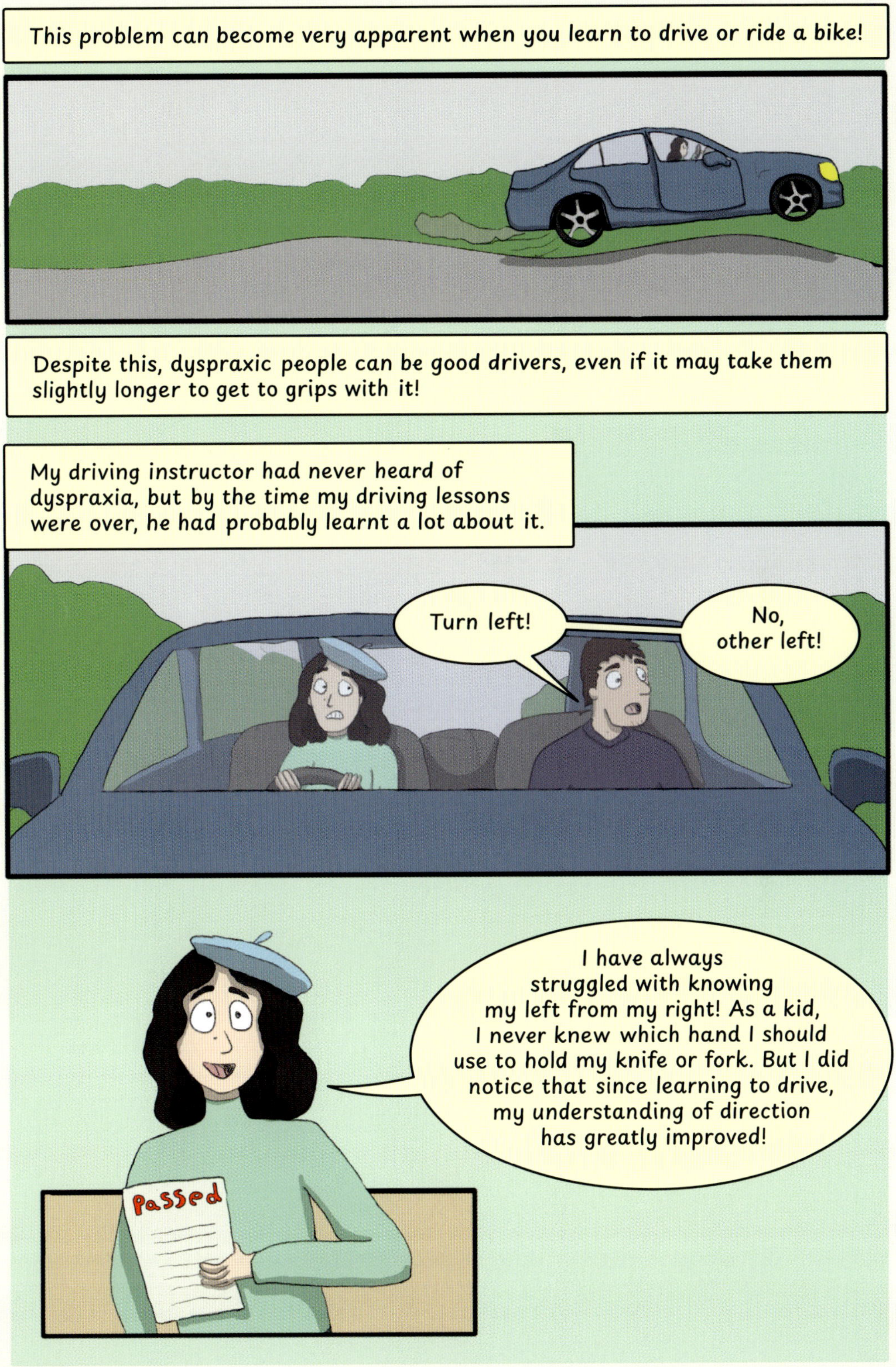
This problem can become very apparent when you learn to drive or ride a bike!
Despite this, dyspraxic people can be good drivers, even if it may take them slightly longer to get to grips with it!
My driving instructor had never heard of dyspraxia, but by the time my driving lessons were over, he had probably learnt a lot about it.
Turn left!
No, other left!
I have always struggled with knowing my left from my right! As a kid, I never knew which hand I should use to hold my knife or fork. But I did notice that since learning to drive, my understanding of direction has greatly improved!
Passed

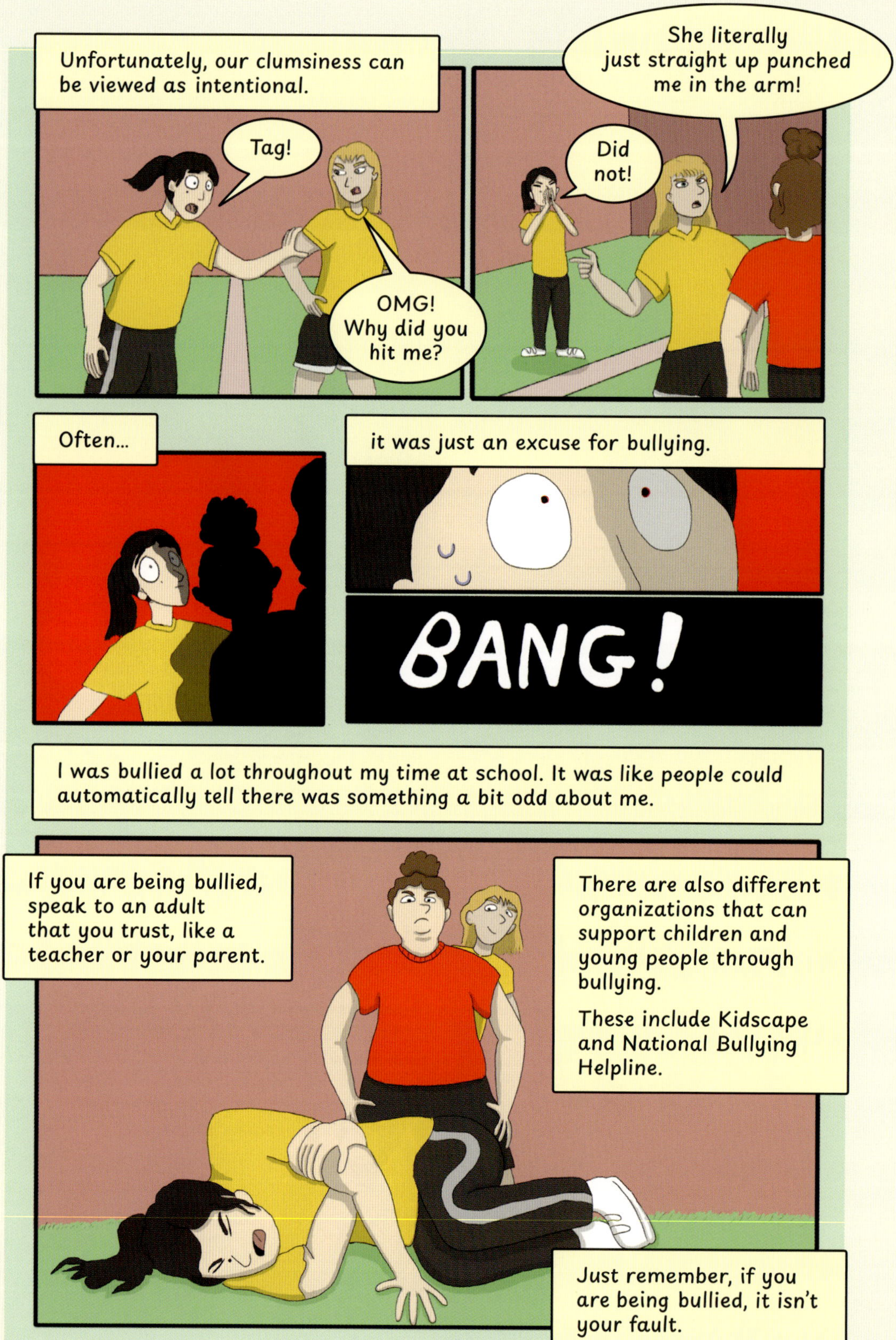
Unfortunately, our clumsiness can be viewed as intentional.
Tag!
OMG! Why did you hit me?
She literally just straight up punched me in the arm!
Did not!
Often...
it was just an excuse for bullying.
BANG!
I was bullied a lot throughout my time at school. It was like people could automatically tell there was something a bit odd about me.
If you are being bullied, speak to an adult that you trust, like a teacher or your parent.
There are also different organizations that can support children and young people through bullying.
These include Kidscape and National Bullying Helpline.
Just remember, if you are being bullied, it isn't your fault.

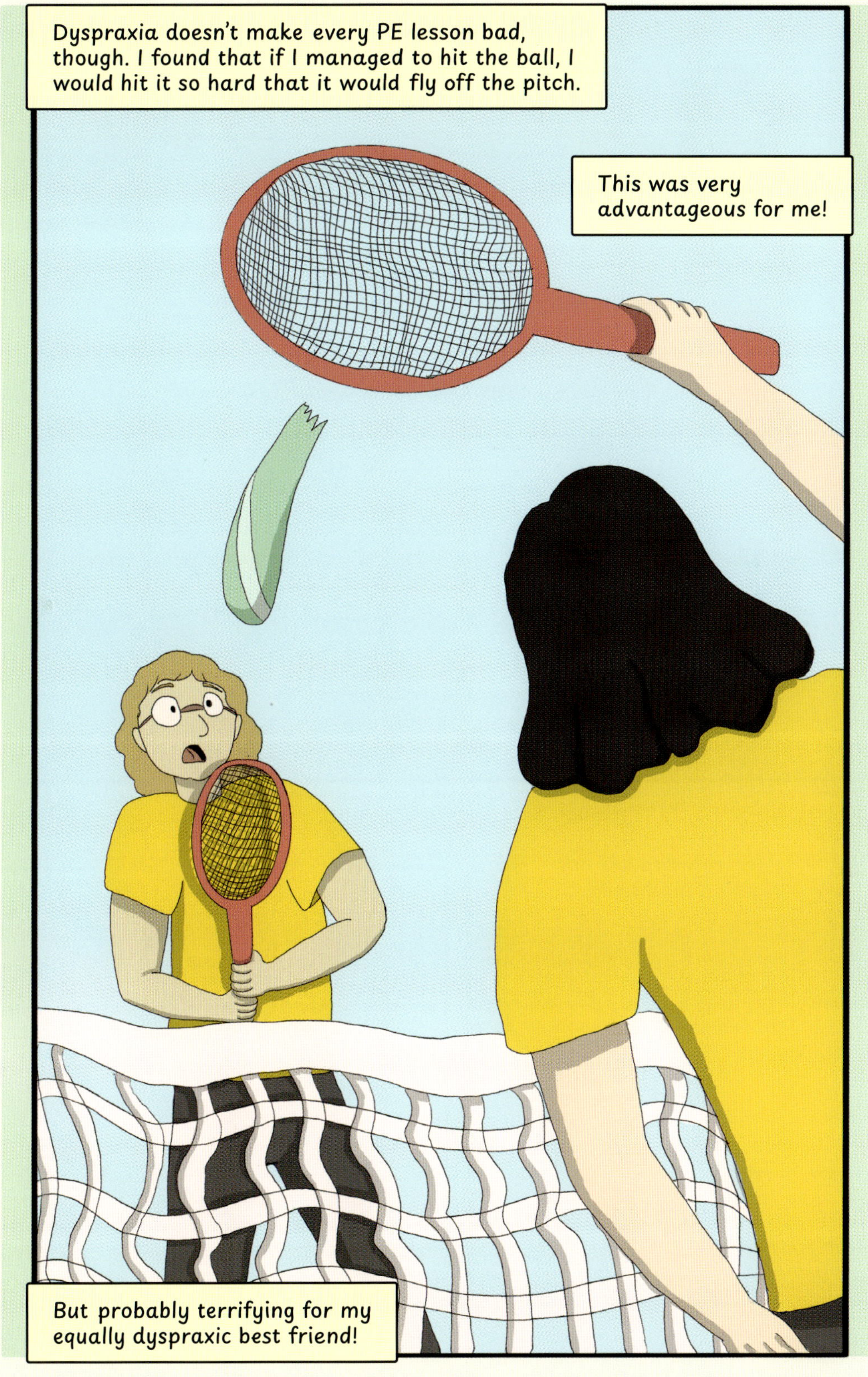
Dyspraxia doesn't make every PE lesson bad, though. I found that if I managed to hit the ball, I would hit it so hard that it would fly off the pitch.
This was very advantageous for me!
But probably terrifying for my equally dyspraxic best friend!

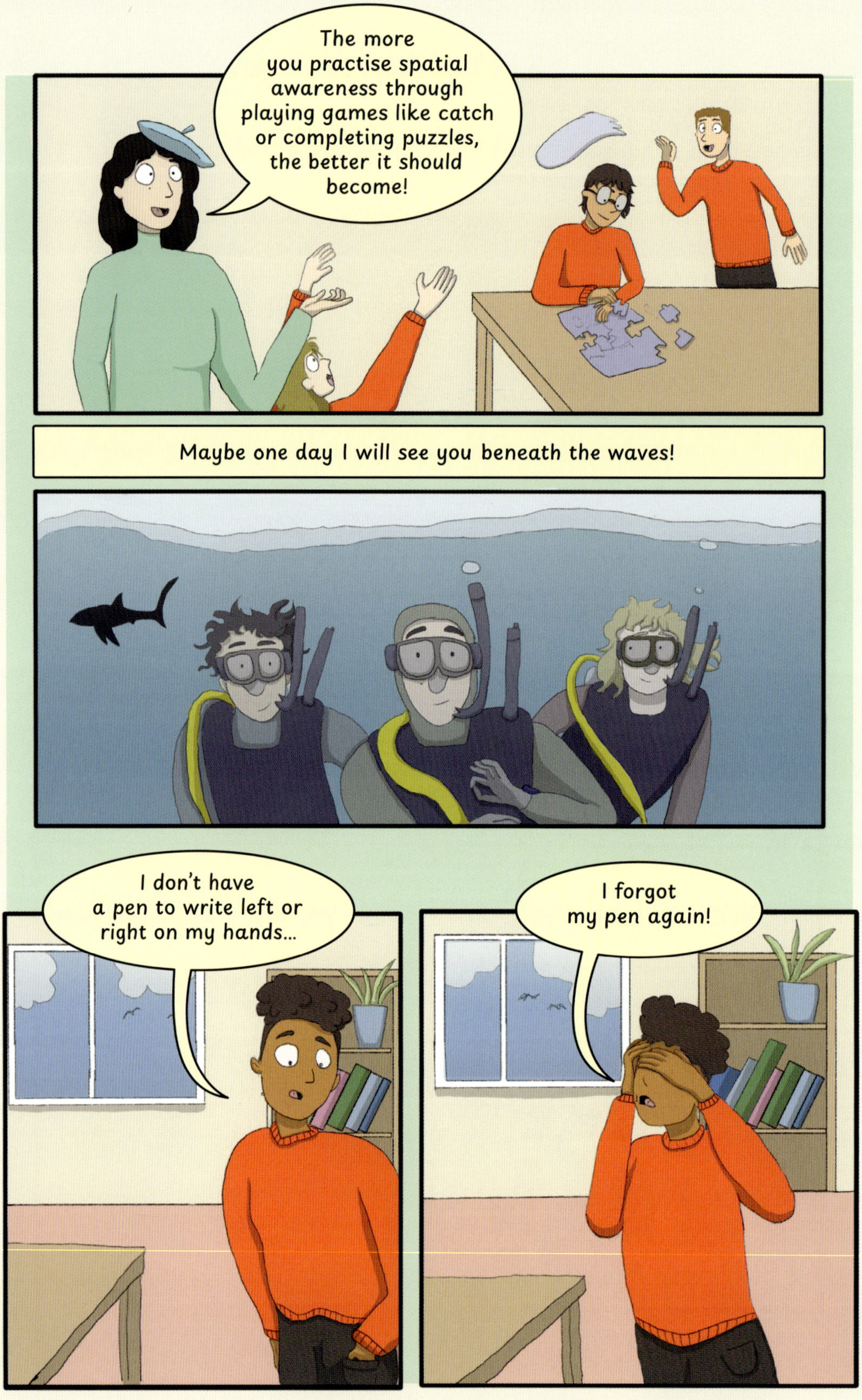
The more you practise spatial awareness through playing games like catch or completing puzzles, the better it should become!
Maybe one day I will see you beneath the waves!
I don't have a pen to write left or right on my hands...
I forgot my pen again!

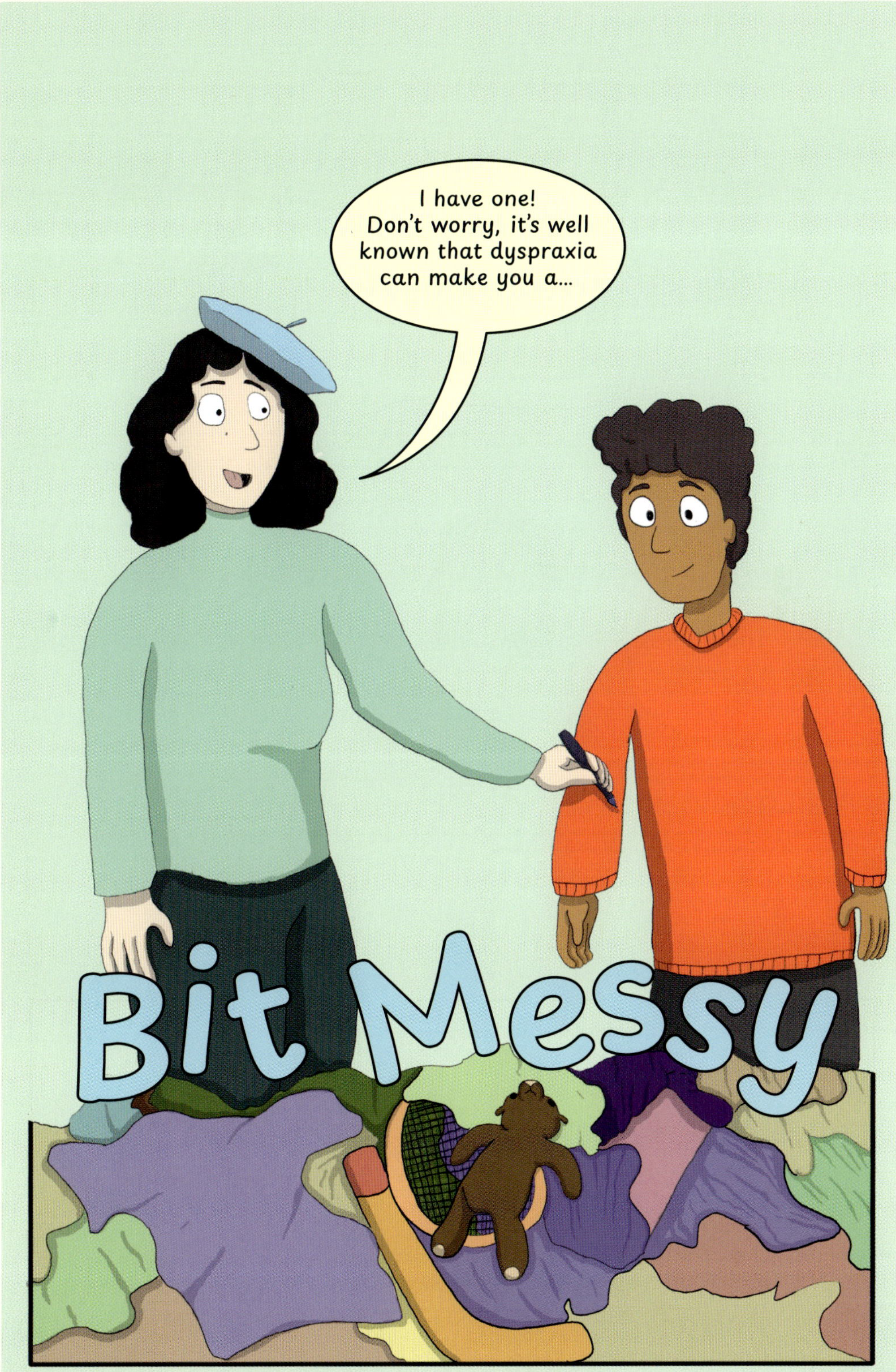
I have one! Don't worry, it's well known that dyspraxia can make you a...
Bit Messy

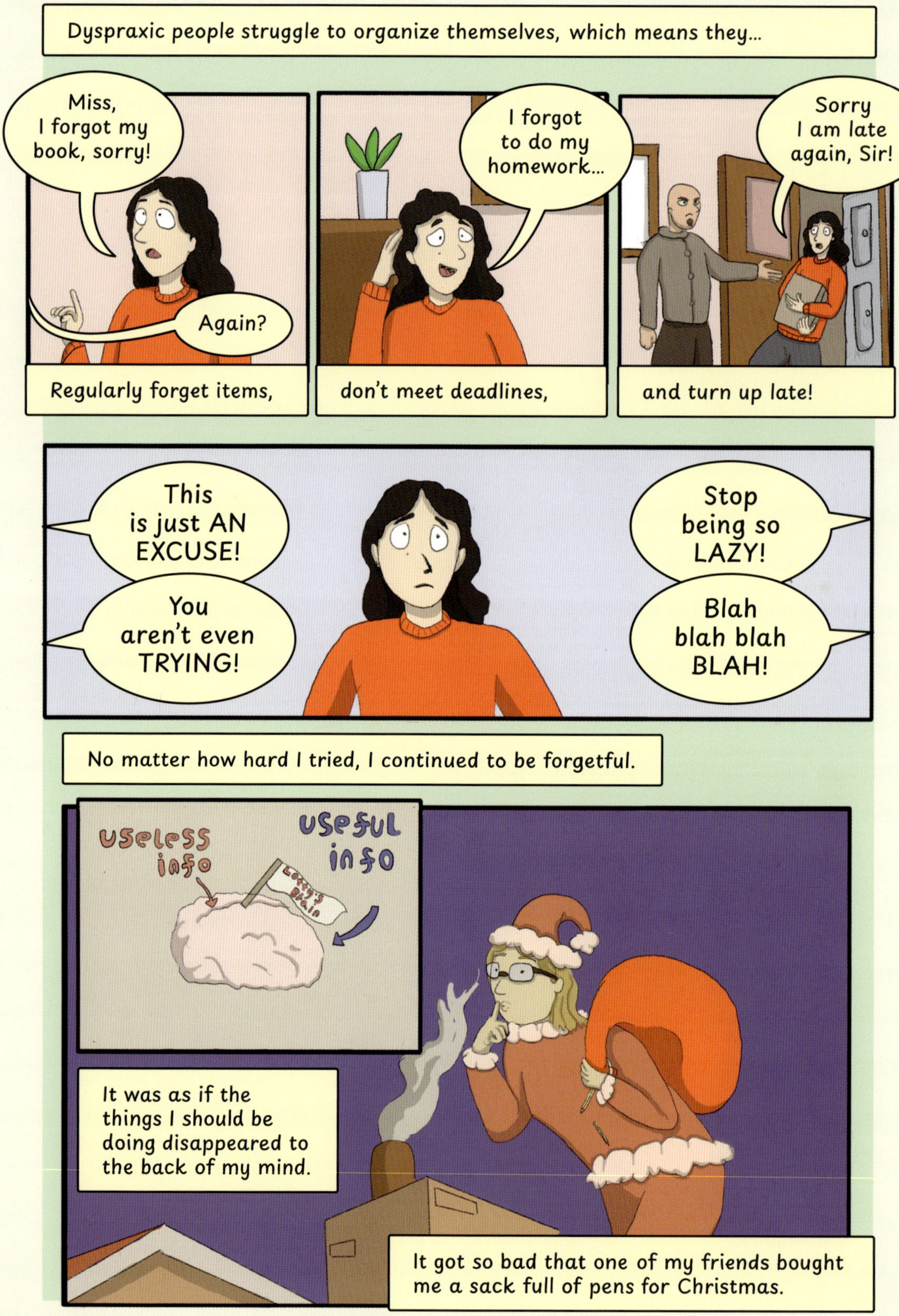

Dyspraxic people struggle to organize themselves, which means they...
Miss, I forgot my book, sorry!
Again?
Regularly forget items,
I forgot to do my homework...
don't meet deadlines,
Sorry I am late again, Sir!
and turn up late!
This is just AN EXCUSE!
You aren't even TRYING!
Stop being so LAZY!
Blah blah blah BLAH!
No matter how hard I tried, I continued to be forgetful.
useless info
useful info
It was as if the things I should be doing disappeared to the back of my mind.
It got so bad that one of my friends bought me a sack full of pens for Christmas.

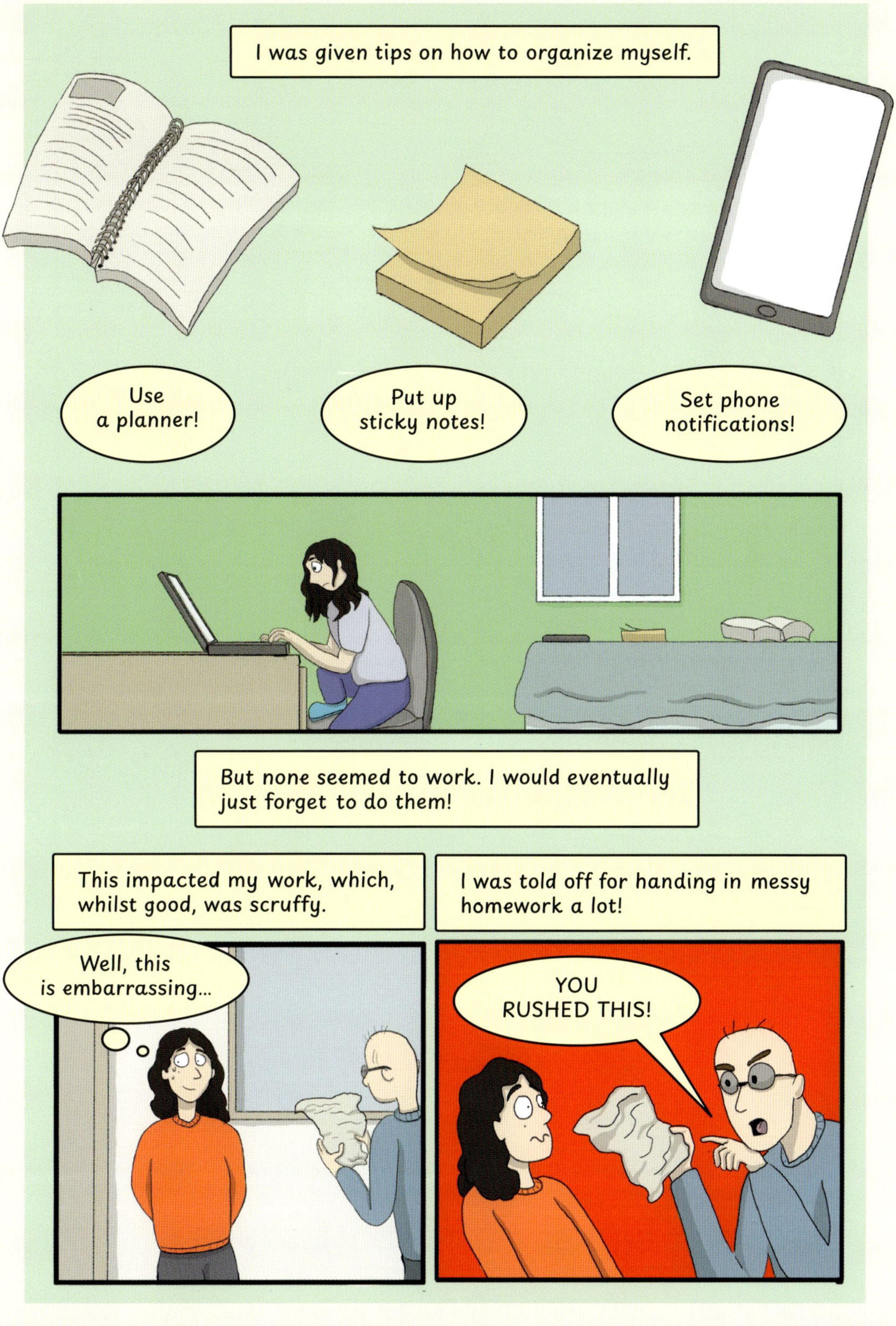

I was given tips on how to organize myself.
Use a planner!
Put up sticky notes!
Set phone notifications!
But none seemed to work. I would eventually just forget to do them!
This impacted my work, which, whilst good, was scruffy.
Well, this is embarrassing...
I was told off for handing in messy homework a lot!
YOU RUSHED THIS!

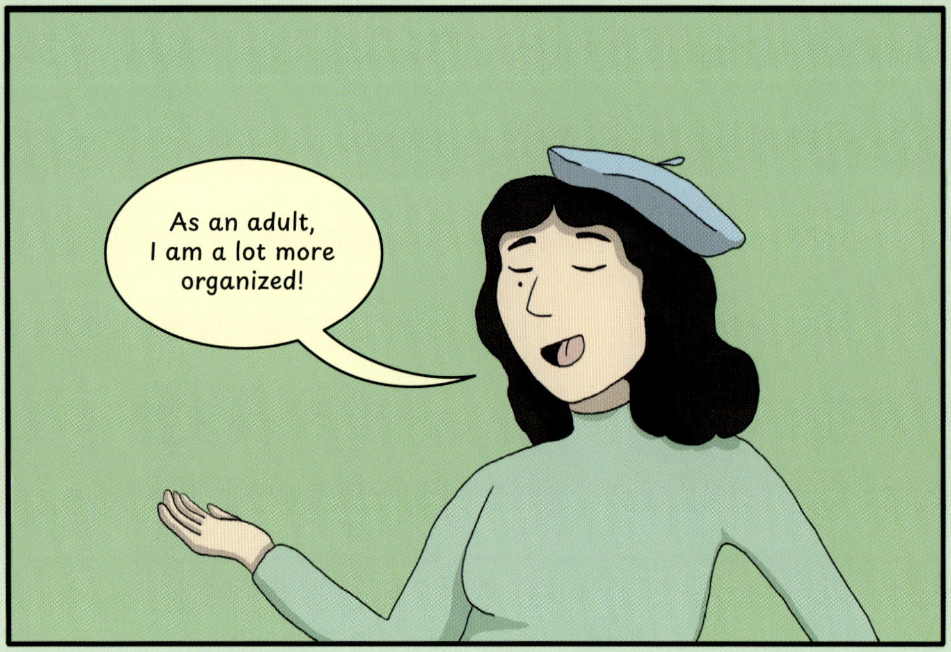
As an adult, I am a lot more organized!

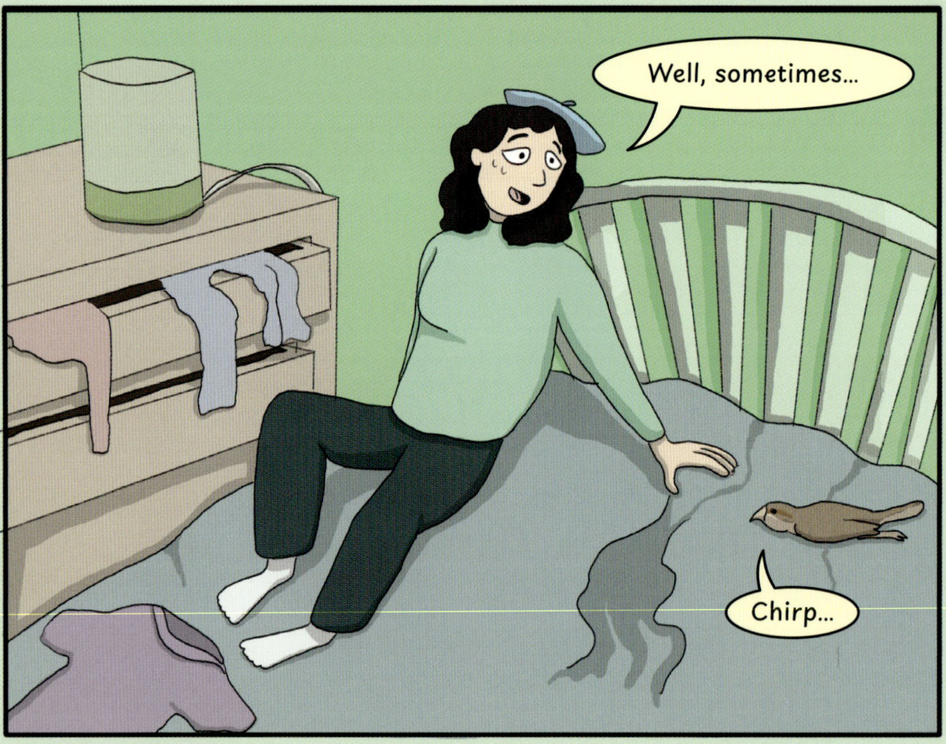
Well, sometimes...
Chirp...

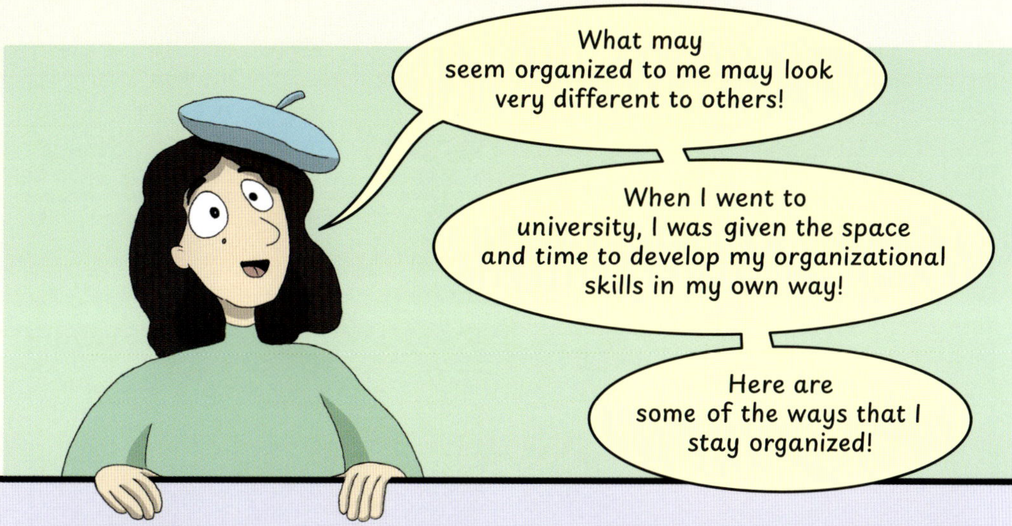
What may seem organized to me may look very different to others!
When I went to university, I was given the space and time to develop my organizational skills in my own way!
Here are some of the ways that I stay organized!

Lotty's top tips for staying organized!

- Make writing in your planner a routine at the end of every school day. It doesn't matter what you write. Just the act of writing daily will make it a habit.
- Make it a routine to look at your planner when you finish school.
- Make sure you pack your school bag the evening before you go to school.
- Write everything you need on a list and make sure you have everything before you leave home.
- Leave in time to get to places 15 minutes before you need to.

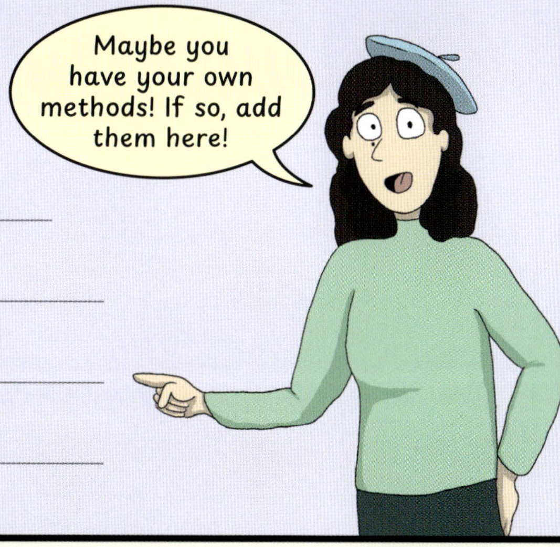
Maybe you have your own methods! If so, add them here!

- ______________________________
- ______________________________
- ______________________________
- ______________________________
- ______________________________

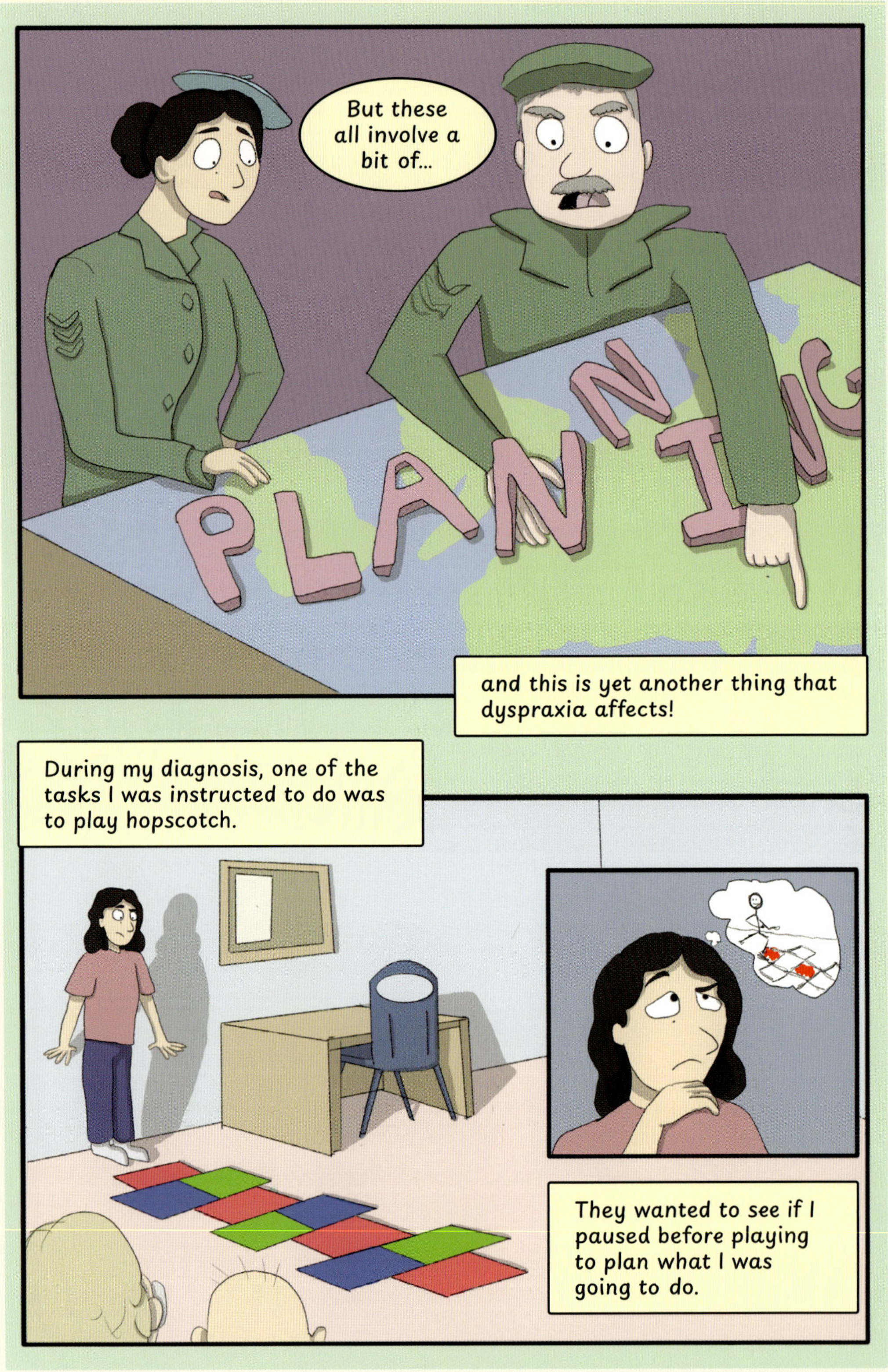
But these all involve a bit of...
PLANNING
and this is yet another thing that dyspraxia affects!
During my diagnosis, one of the tasks I was instructed to do was to play hopscotch.
They wanted to see if I paused before playing to plan what I was going to do.

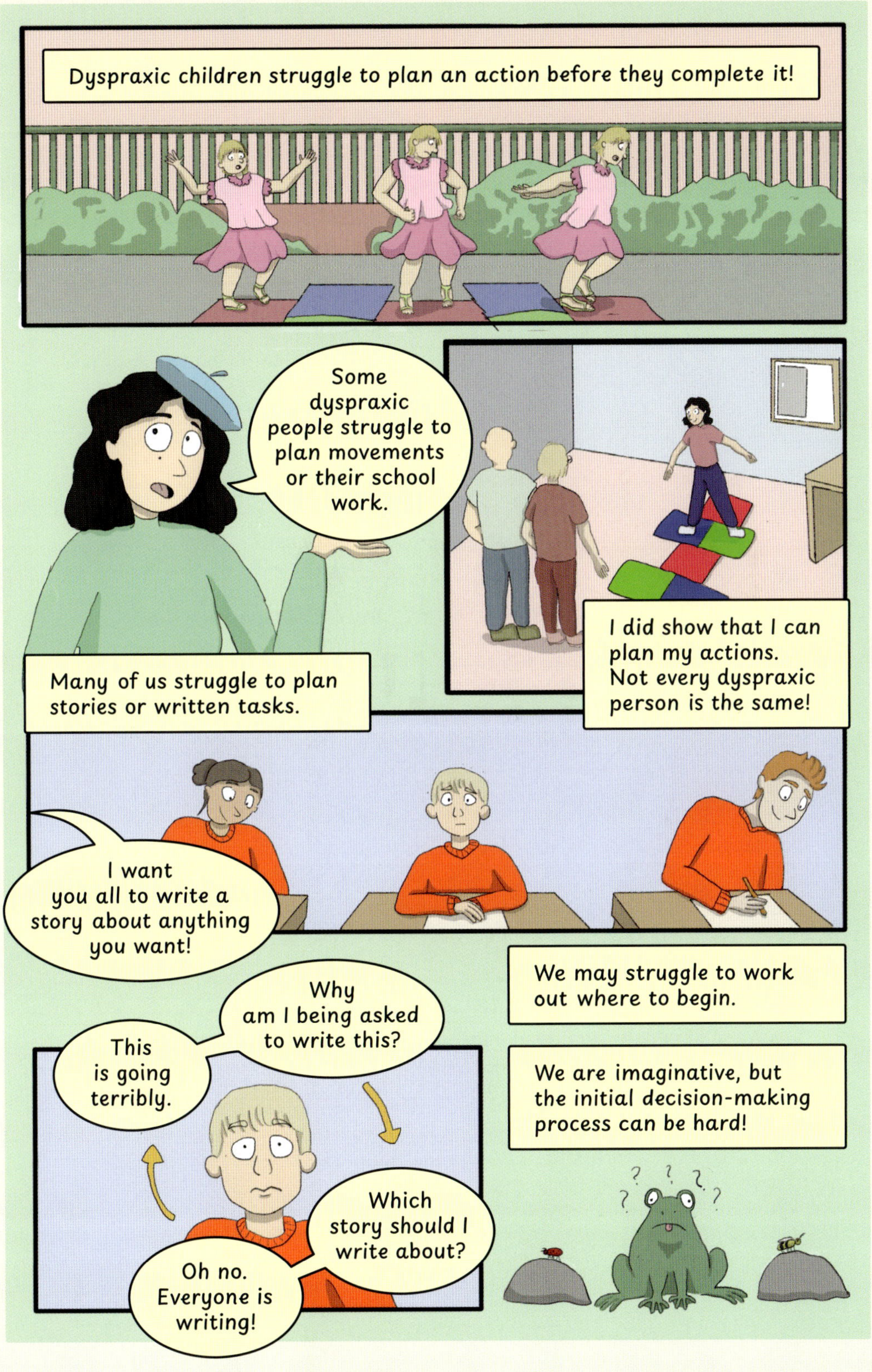

Dyspraxic children struggle to plan an action before they complete it!
Some dyspraxic people struggle to plan movements or their school work.
Many of us struggle to plan stories or written tasks.
I did show that I can plan my actions. Not every dyspraxic person is the same!
I want you all to write a story about anything you want!
We may struggle to work out where to begin.
Why am I being asked to write this?
This is going terribly.
Which story should I write about?
Oh no. Everyone is writing!
We are imaginative, but the initial decision-making process can be hard!

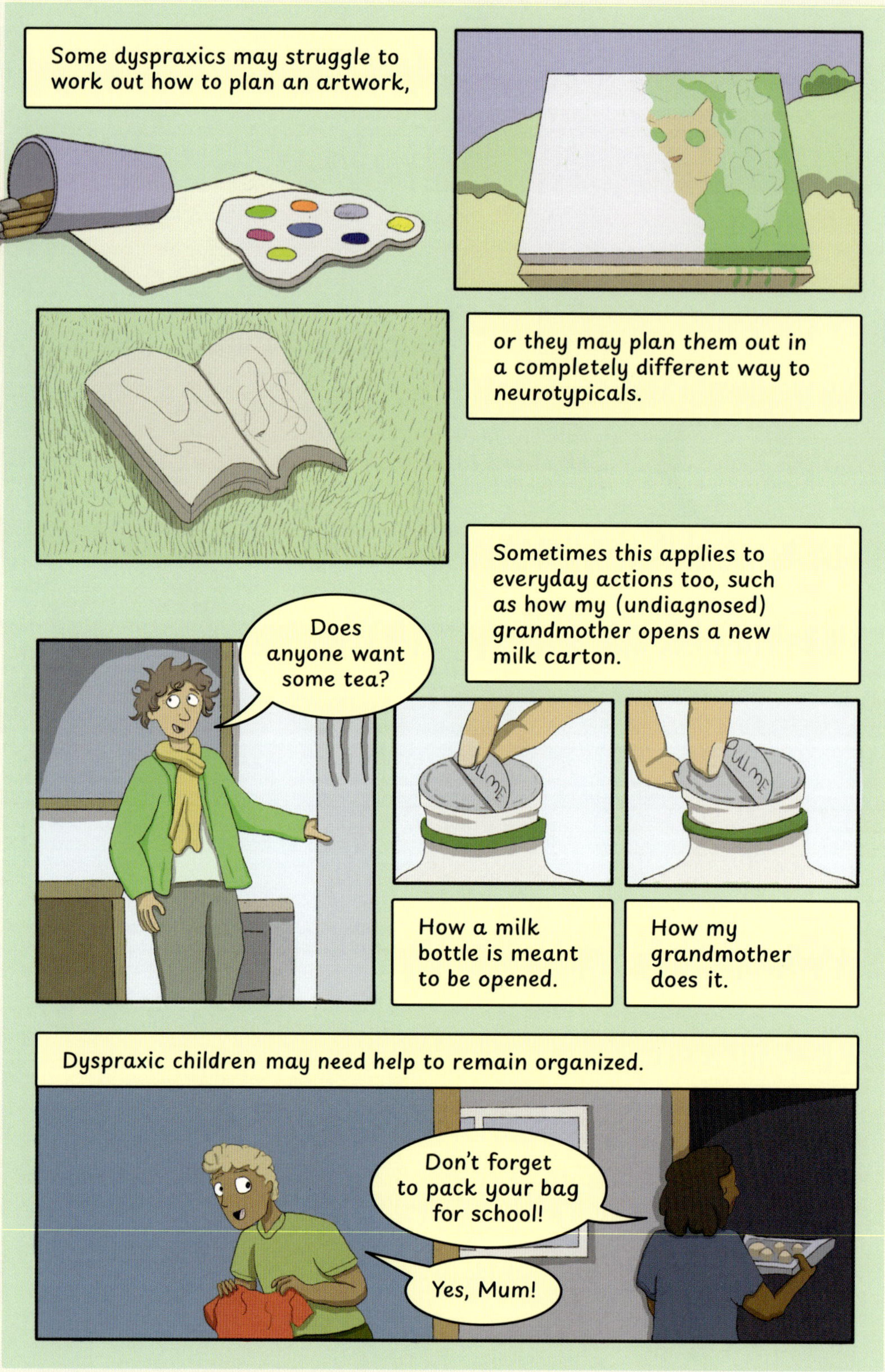
Some dyspraxics may struggle to work out how to plan an artwork,
or they may plan them out in a completely different way to neurotypicals.
Sometimes this applies to everyday actions too, such as how my (undiagnosed) grandmother opens a new milk carton.
Does anyone want some tea?
How a milk bottle is meant to be opened.
How my grandmother does it.
Dyspraxic children may need help to remain organized.
Don't forget to pack your bag for school!
Yes, Mum!

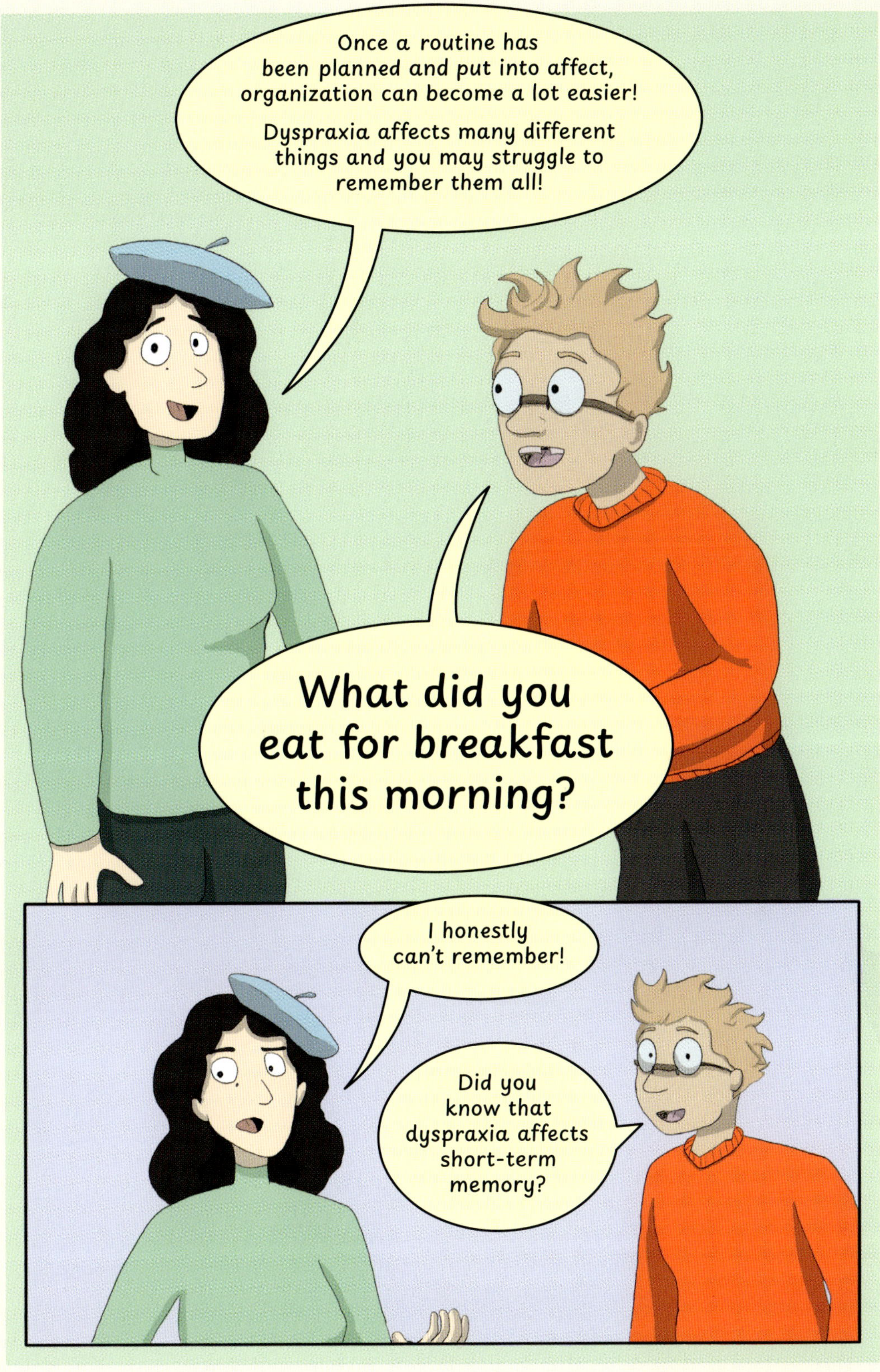
Once a routine has been planned and put into affect, organization can become a lot easier!
Dyspraxia affects many different things and you may struggle to remember them all!
What did you eat for breakfast this morning?
I honestly can't remember!
Did you know that dyspraxia affects short-term memory?

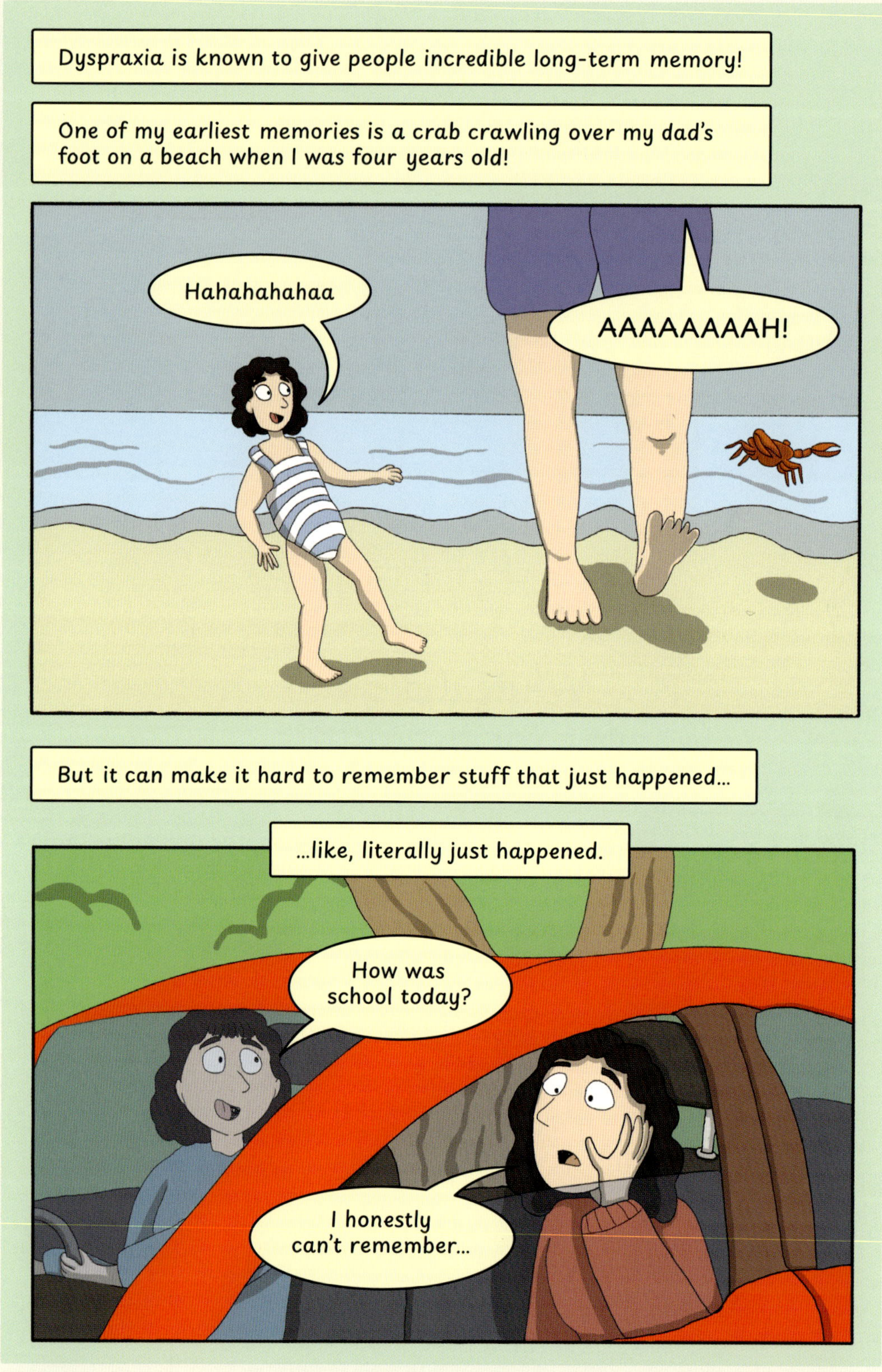
Dyspraxia is known to give people incredible long-term memory!
One of my earliest memories is a crab crawling over my dad's foot on a beach when I was four years old!
Hahahahahaa
AAAAAAAAH!
But it can make it hard to remember stuff that just happened...
...like, literally just happened.
How was school today?
I honestly can't remember...

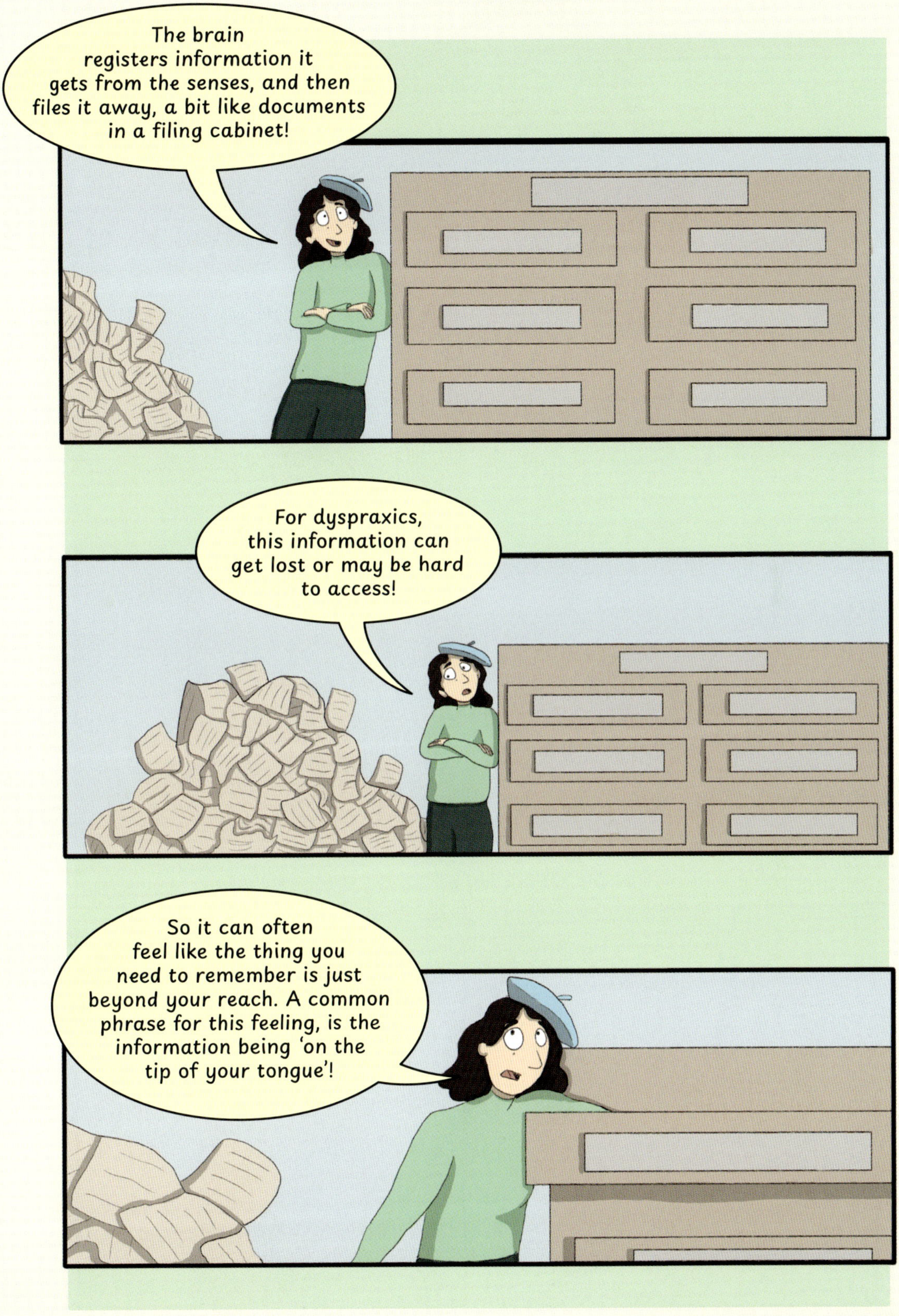

The brain registers information it gets from the senses, and then files it away, a bit like documents in a filing cabinet!
For dyspraxics, this information can get lost or may be hard to access!
So it can often feel like the thing you need to remember is just beyond your reach. A common phrase for this feeling, is the information being 'on the tip of your tongue'!

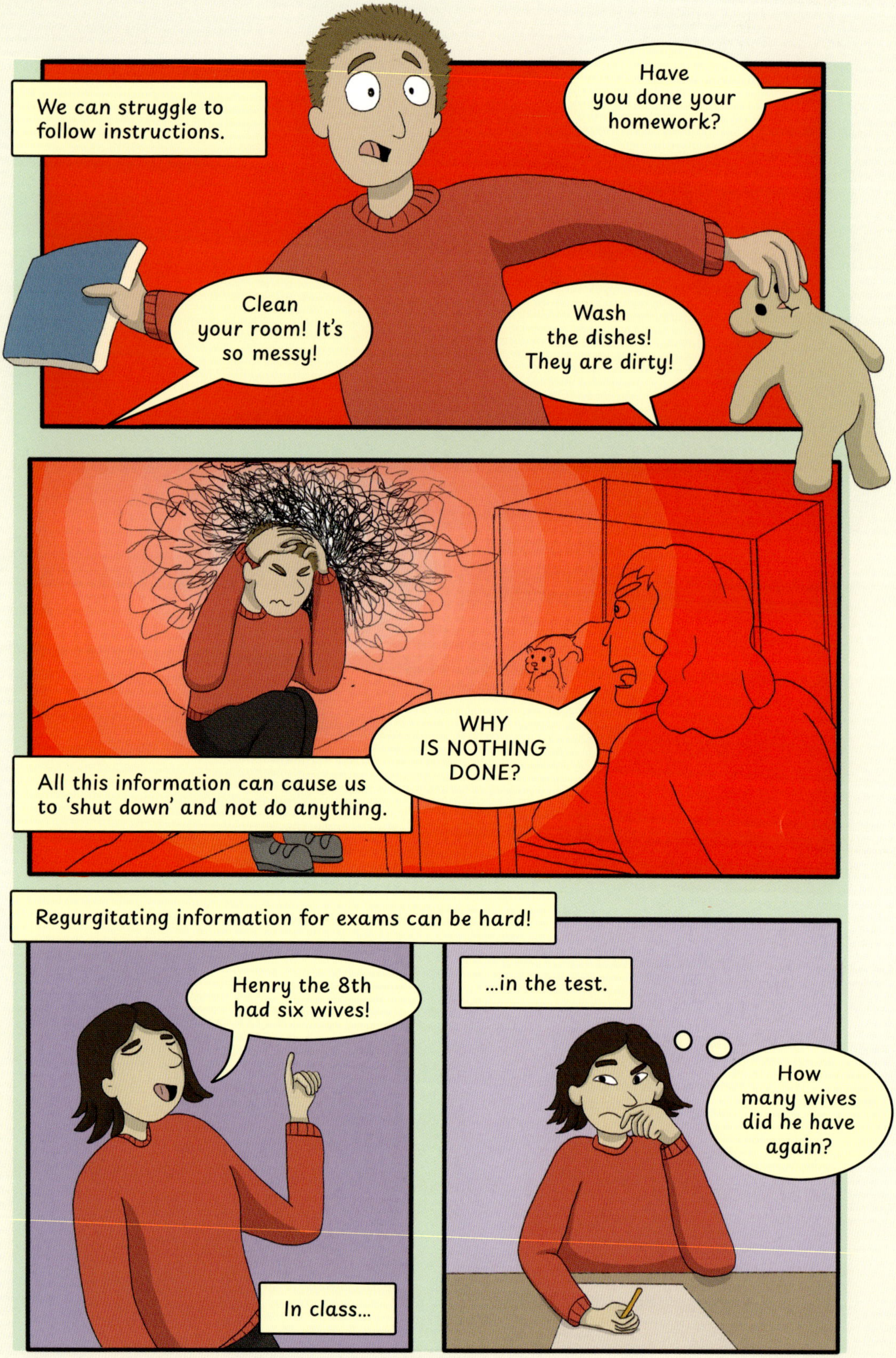
We can struggle to follow instructions.
Have you done your homework?
Clean your room! It's so messy!
Wash the dishes! They are dirty!
All this information can cause us to 'shut down' and not do anything.
WHY IS NOTHING DONE?
Regurgitating information for exams can be hard!
Henry the 8th had six wives!
In class...
...in the test.
How many wives did he have again?

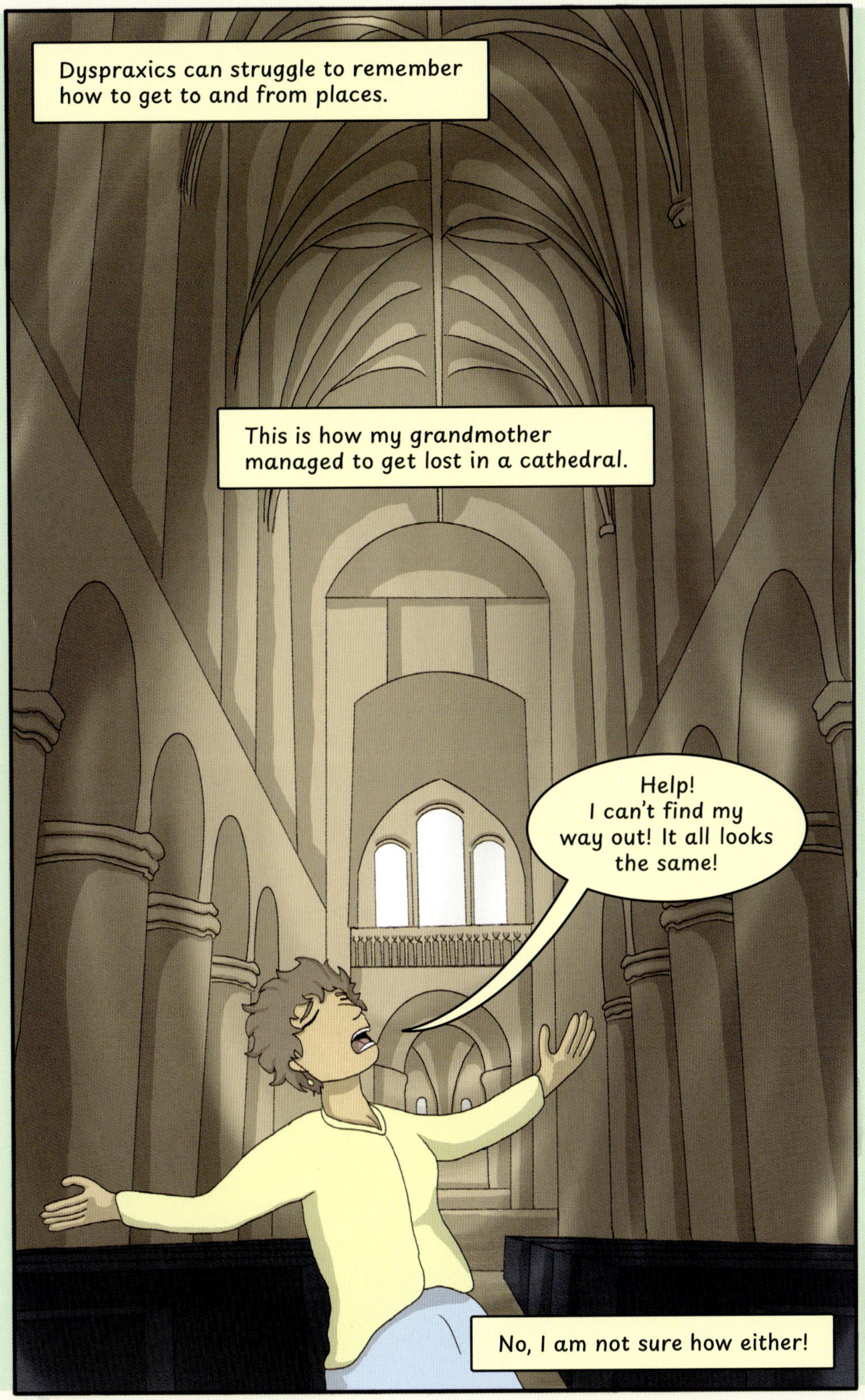
Dyspraxics can struggle to remember how to get to and from places.
This is how my grandmother managed to get lost in a cathedral.
Help! I can't find my way out! It all looks the same!
No, I am not sure how either!

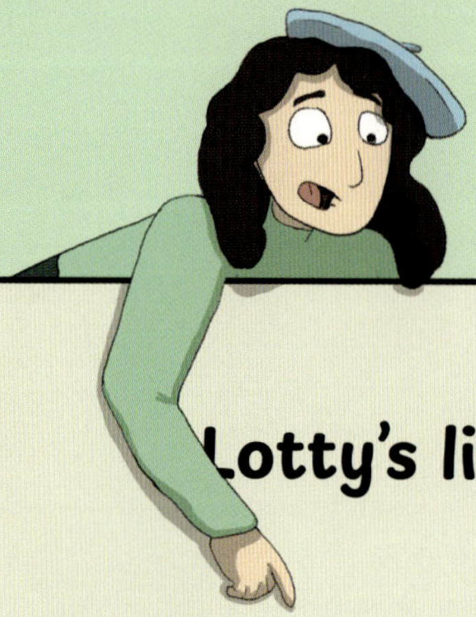

Lotty's list to remember!

- Repeating a task over and over can help to secure a memory, making it easier to remember. This can help in tasks like driving or learning how to ride a bike, where the same actions are repeated.
- Similarly, revising words and explaining ideas to people or yourself repeatedly can help you to remember them. Dyspraxic people may need to do this a few more times than their classmates, but it works!
- Writing down words that can link to a fact or thing you need to remember, or just writing down what needs to be remembered can also be helpful and save embarrassment.
- As I have said before, get into the routine of writing things down in a journal and checking it at the end of the day. This will ensure that you don't accidentally forget something that you are meant to do.

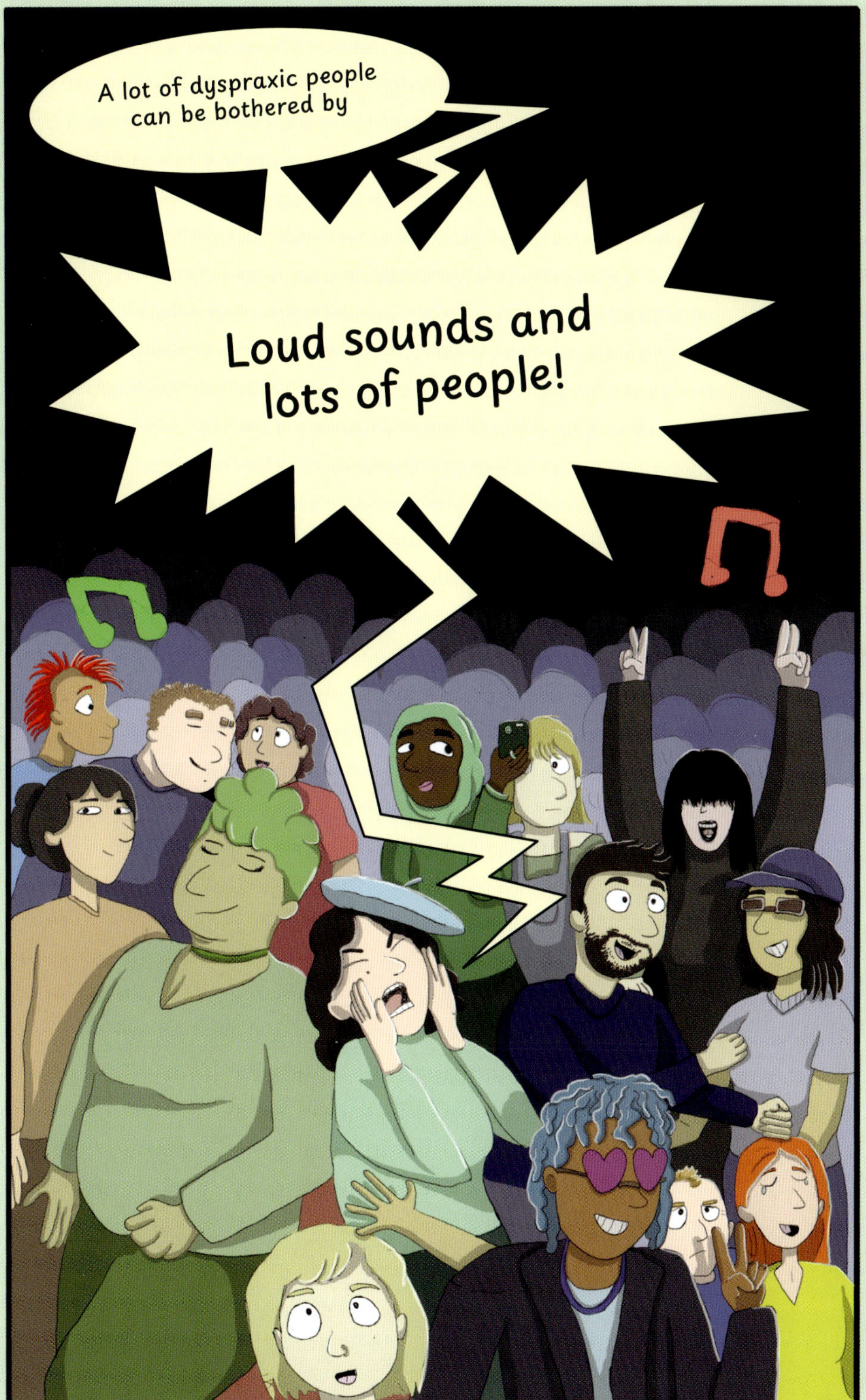
A lot of dyspraxic people can be bothered by
Loud sounds and lots of people!

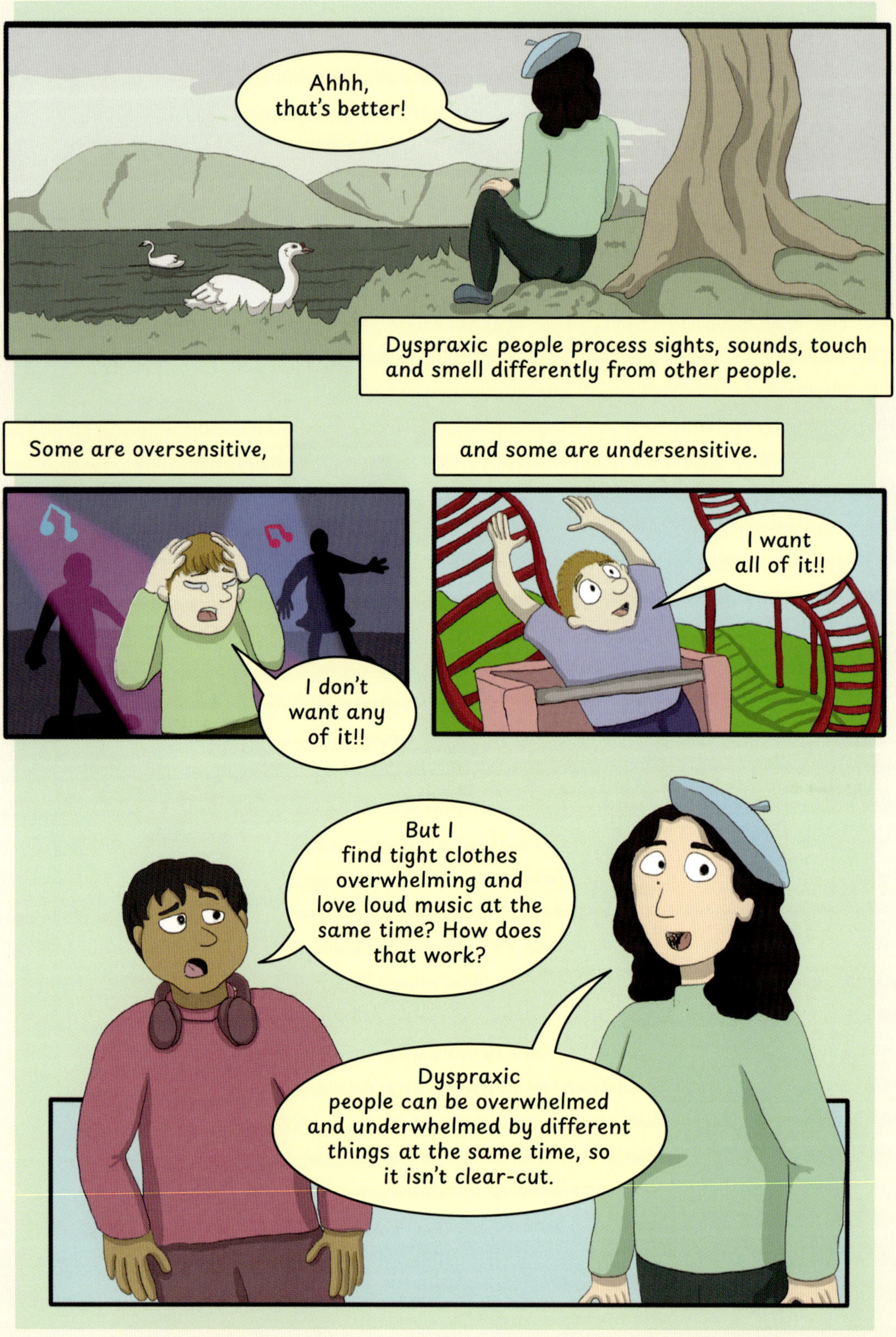
Ahhh, that's better!
Dyspraxic people process sights, sounds, touch and smell differently from other people.
Some are oversensitive,
and some are undersensitive.
I don't want any of it!!
I want all of it!!
But I find tight clothes overwhelming and love loud music at the same time? How does that work?
Dyspraxic people can be overwhelmed and underwhelmed by different things at the same time, so it isn't clear-cut.

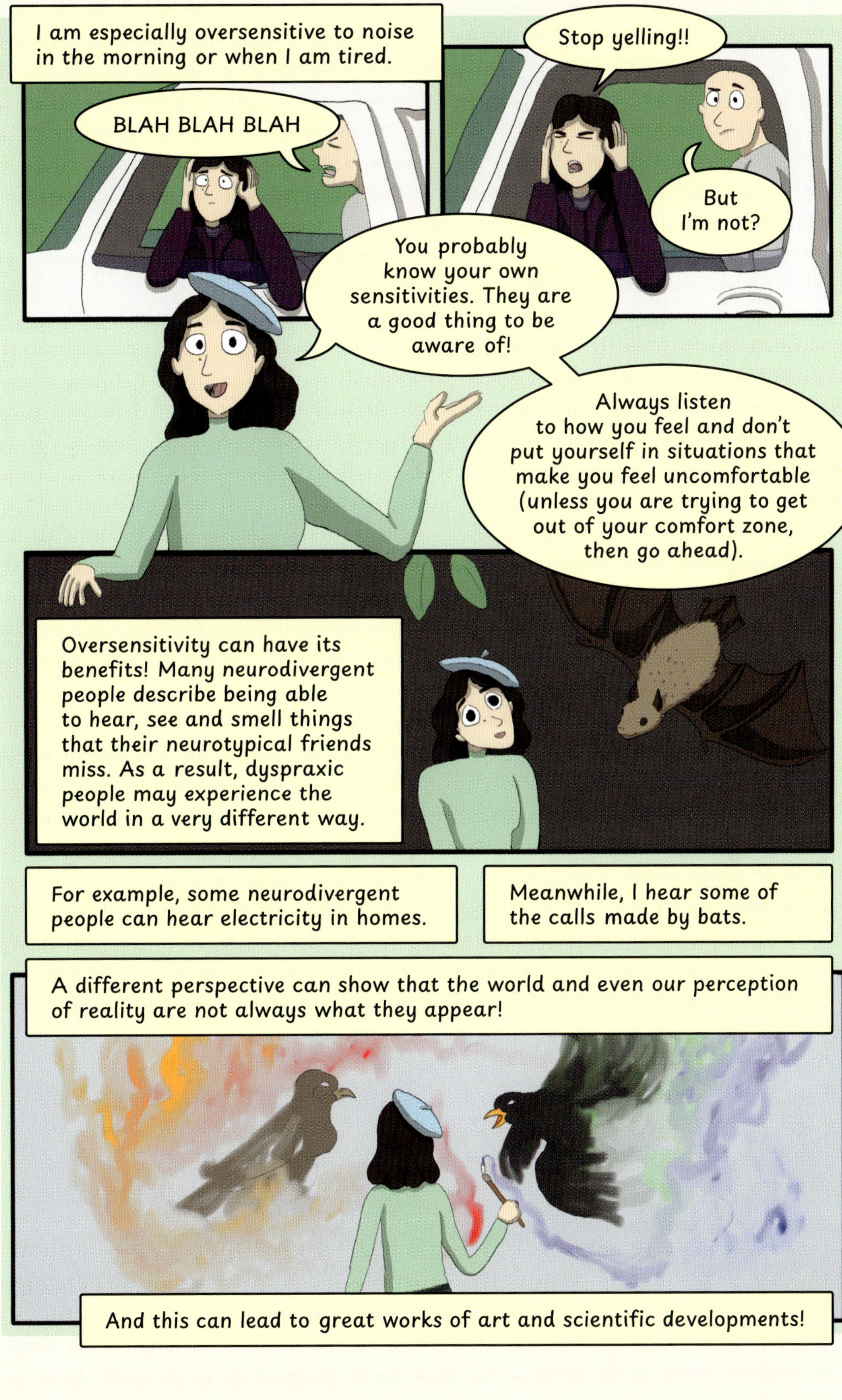
I am especially oversensitive to noise in the morning or when I am tired.
BLAH BLAH BLAH
Stop yelling!!
But I'm not?
You probably know your own sensitivities. They are a good thing to be aware of!
Always listen to how you feel and don't put yourself in situations that make you feel uncomfortable (unless you are trying to get out of your comfort zone, then go ahead).
Oversensitivity can have its benefits! Many neurodivergent people describe being able to hear, see and smell things that their neurotypical friends miss. As a result, dyspraxic people may experience the world in a very different way.
For example, some neurodivergent people can hear electricity in homes.
Meanwhile, I hear some of the calls made by bats.
A different perspective can show that the world and even our perception of reality are not always what they appear!
And this can lead to great works of art and scientific developments!

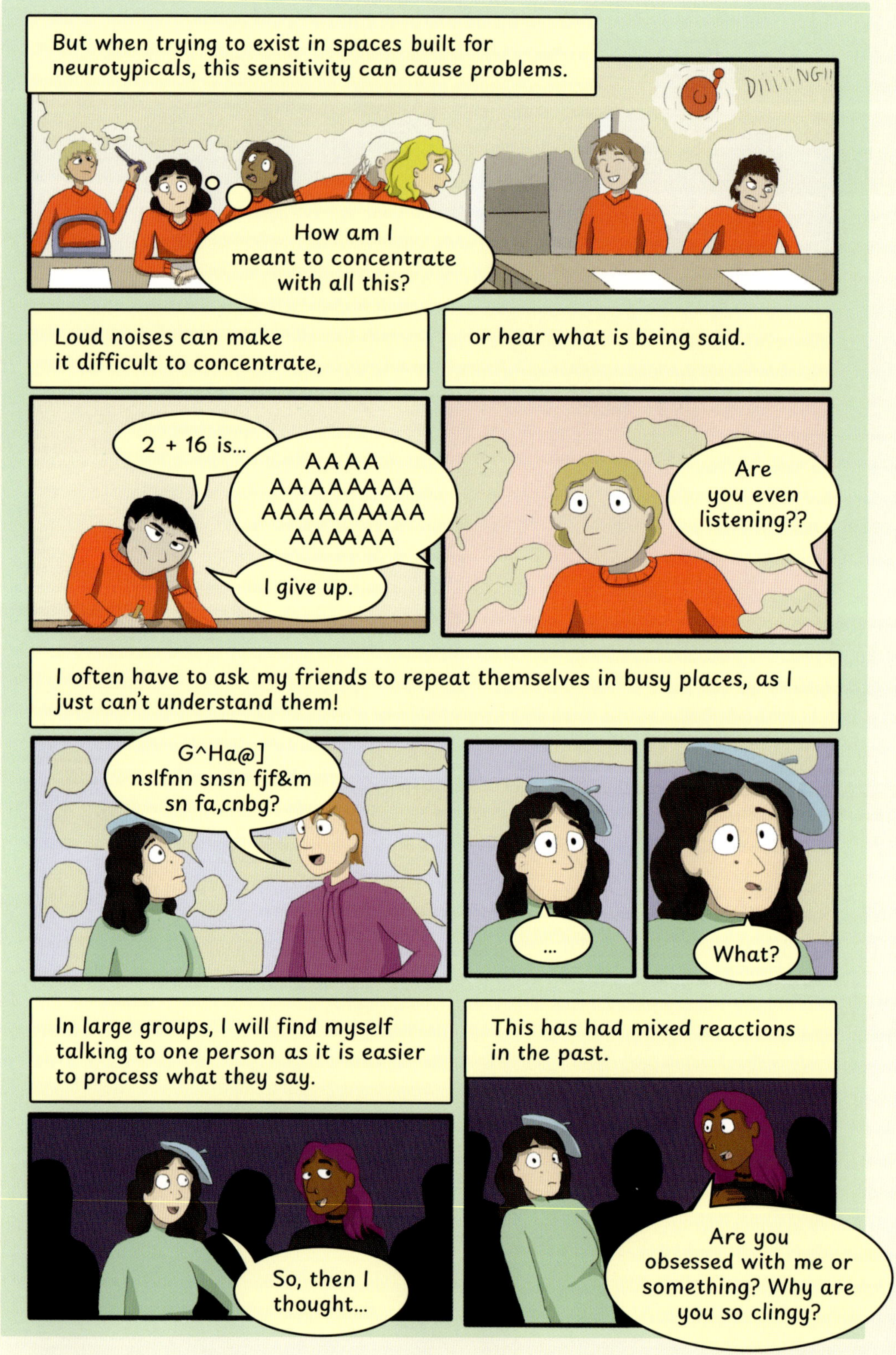

But when trying to exist in spaces built for neurotypicals, this sensitivity can cause problems.
DIIIIING!!
How am I meant to concentrate with all this?
Loud noises can make it difficult to concentrate,
or hear what is being said.
2 + 16 is...
AAAA AAAAAAAA AAAAAAAAA AAAAAA
I give up.
Are you even listening??
I often have to ask my friends to repeat themselves in busy places, as I just can't understand them!
G^Ha@] nslfnn snsn fjf&m sn fa,cnbg?
...
What?
In large groups, I will find myself talking to one person as it is easier to process what they say.
So, then I thought...
This has had mixed reactions in the past.
Are you obsessed with me or something? Why are you so clingy?

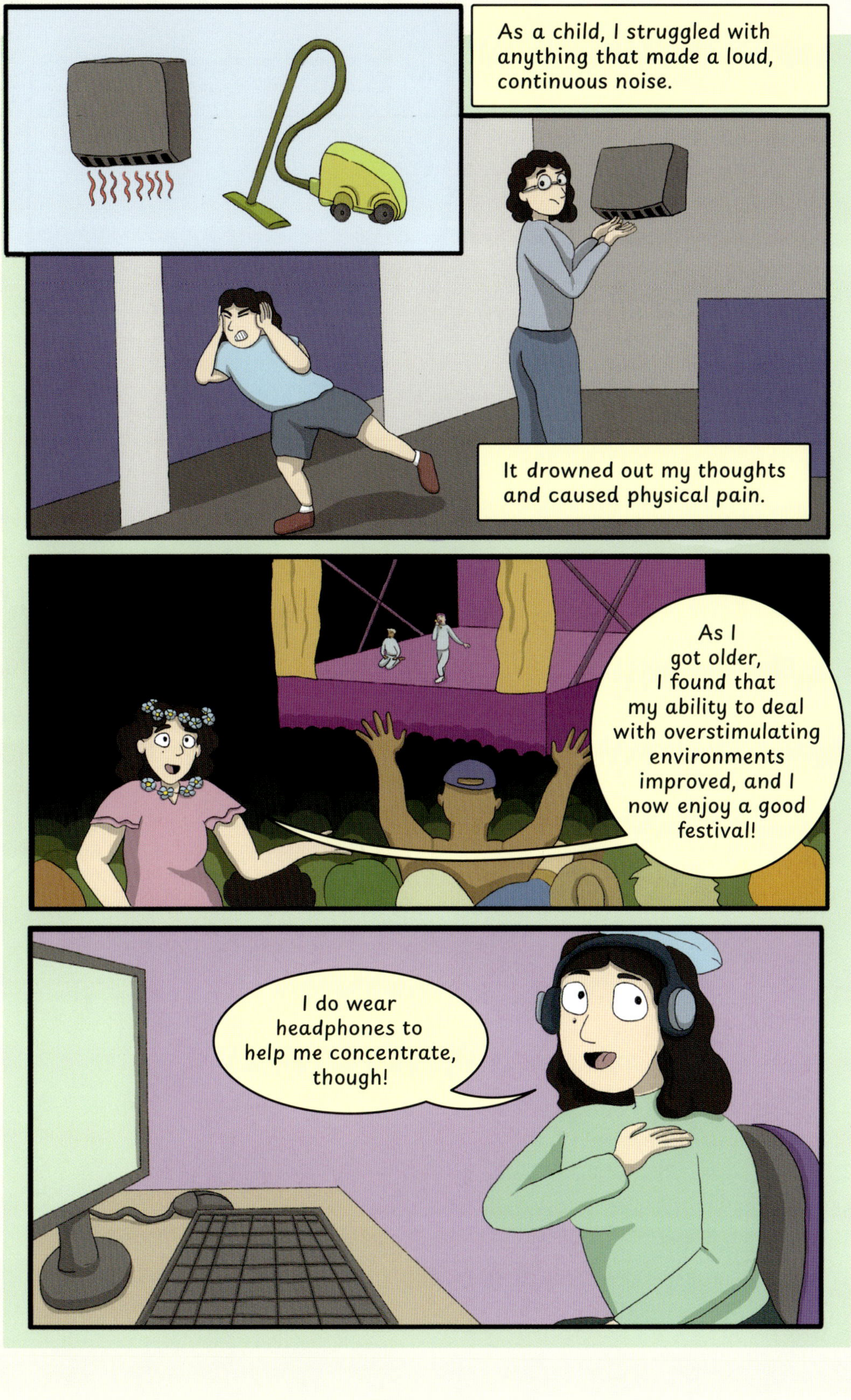
As a child, I struggled with anything that made a loud, continuous noise.
It drowned out my thoughts and caused physical pain.
As I got older, I found that my ability to deal with overstimulating environments improved, and I now enjoy a good festival!
I do wear headphones to help me concentrate, though!

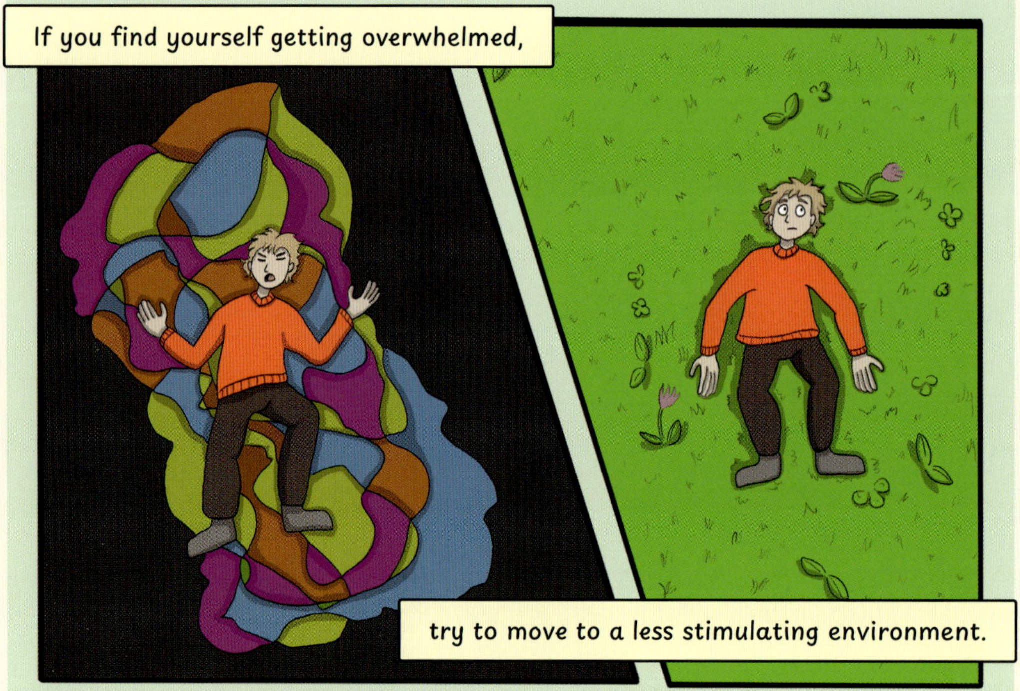
If you find yourself getting overwhelmed,
try to move to a less stimulating environment.

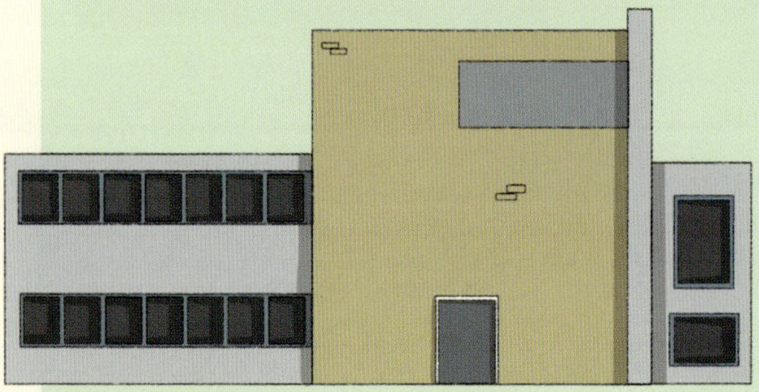

Places like schools and universities often have rooms created specifically to be understimulating.

Ask your school if there are any quiet rooms that you can go to if you are feeling overwhelmed in your classroom or during lunchtime.

As the world is becoming more aware of neurodiversity, other places too often provide spaces for neurodivergent people.

Hospitals often have green spaces that you can access, specifically created for the mental health of patients.

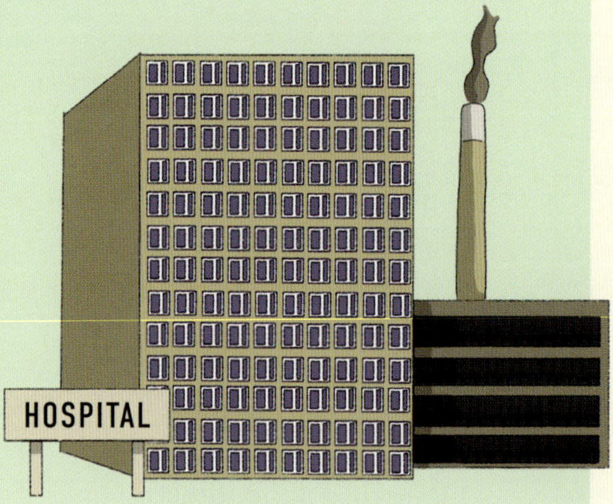

If you require access to a quiet space, the best thing to do is to ask for it. Advocating for yourself is a good way to obtain what you need and may lead to changes that might also benefit others.

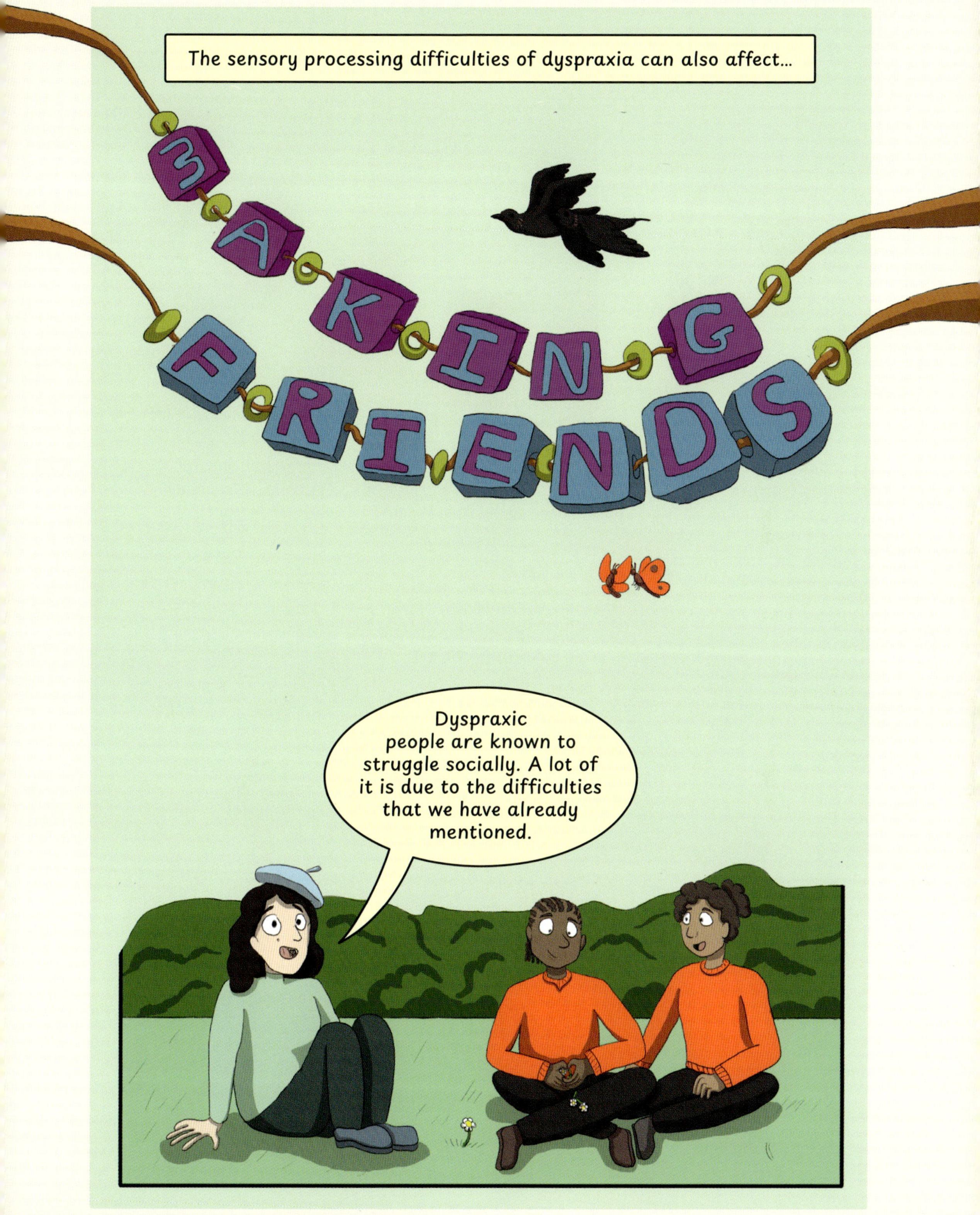
The sensory processing difficulties of dyspraxia can also affect...
MAKING FRIENDS
Dyspraxic people are known to struggle socially. A lot of it is due to the difficulties that we have already mentioned.

Processing difficulties can mean it takes longer for dyspraxic people to respond to a question, or add their own comments to a conversation.

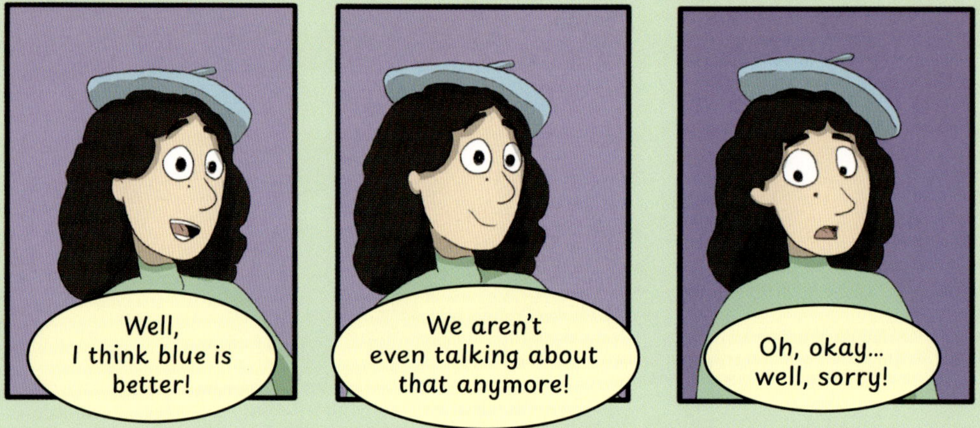

Well, I think blue is better!
We aren't even talking about that anymore!
Oh, okay... well, sorry!

Dyspraxic people are more likely to interrupt too, because they don't understand when to jump in during a conversation. They may also just want to get a thought out before they forget it or the conversation inevitably moves on.

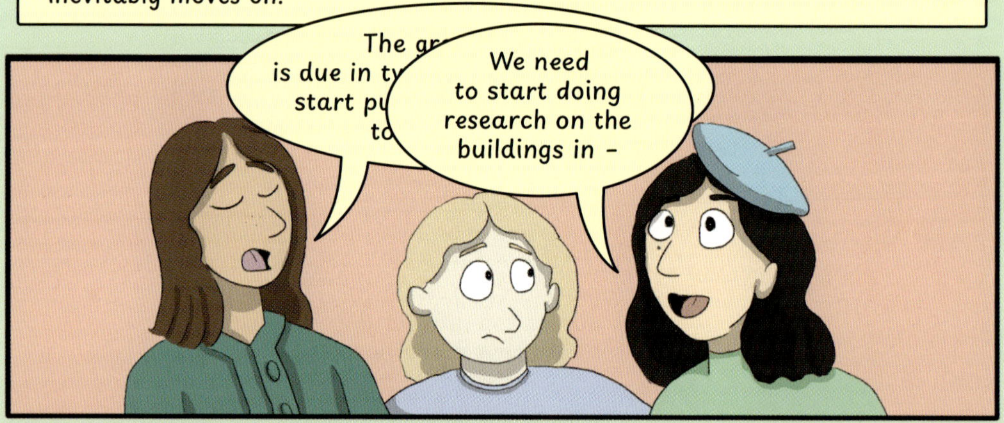

We need to start doing research on the buildings in –

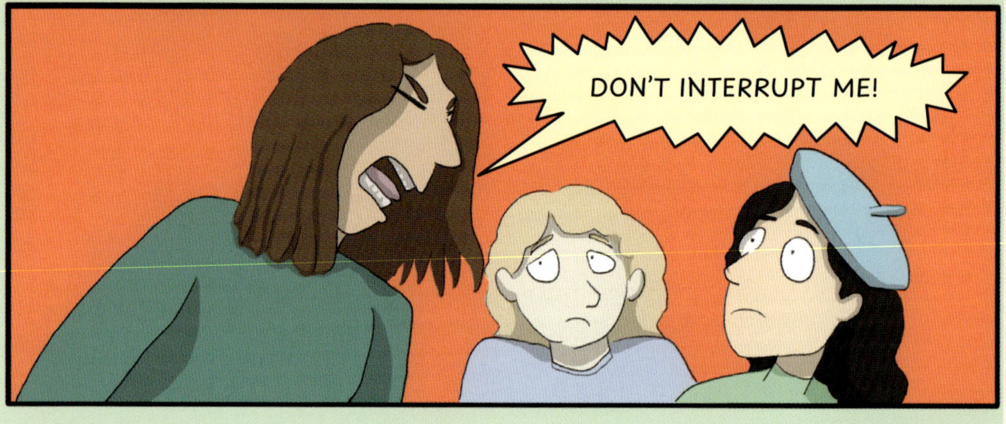

DON'T INTERRUPT ME!

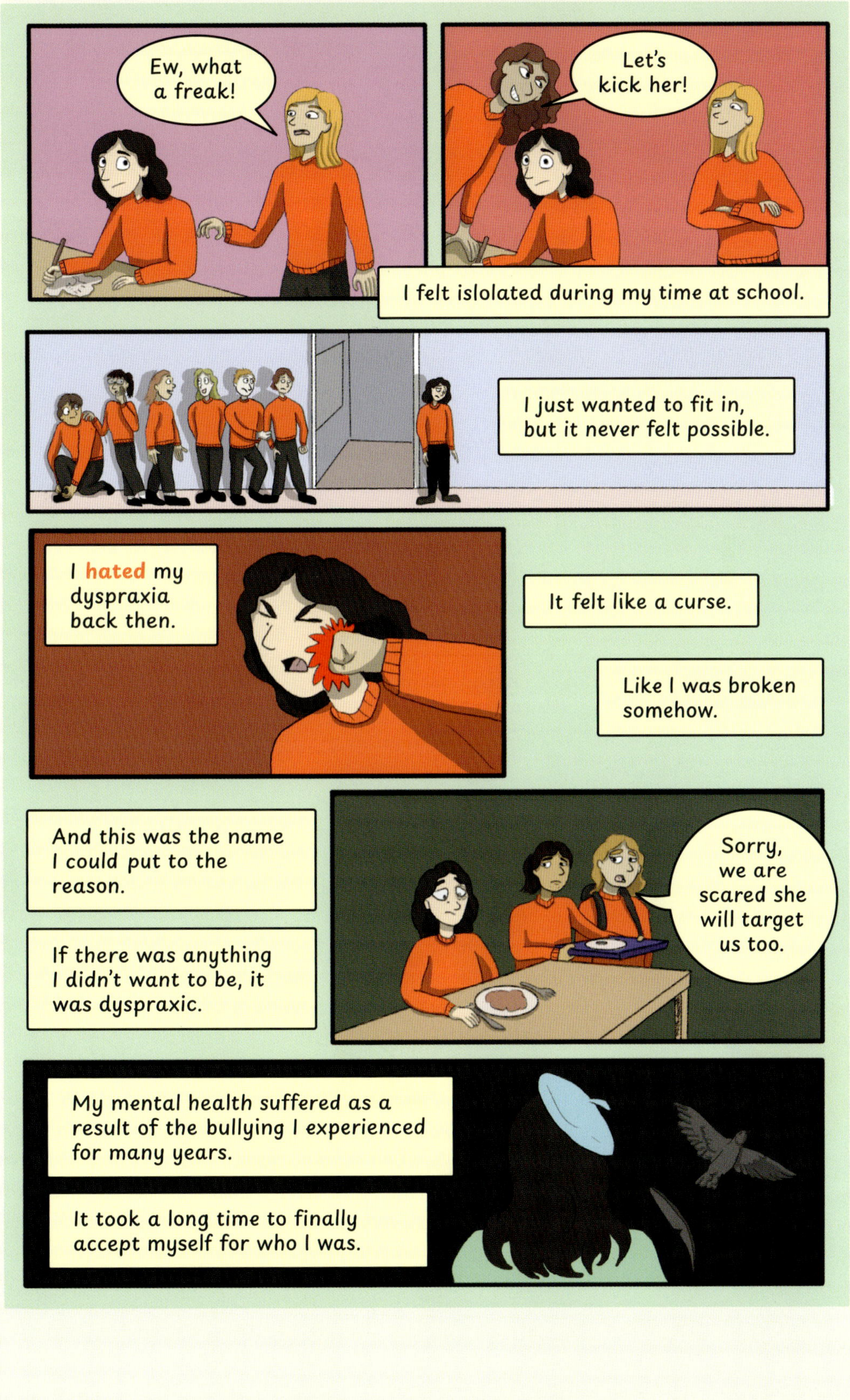

Ew, what a freak!
Let's kick her!
I felt islolated during my time at school.
I just wanted to fit in, but it never felt possible.
I **hated** my dyspraxia back then.
It felt like a curse.
Like I was broken somehow.
And this was the name I could put to the reason.
If there was anything I didn't want to be, it was dyspraxic.
Sorry, we are scared she will target us too.
My mental health suffered as a result of the bullying I experienced for many years.
It took a long time to finally accept myself for who I was.

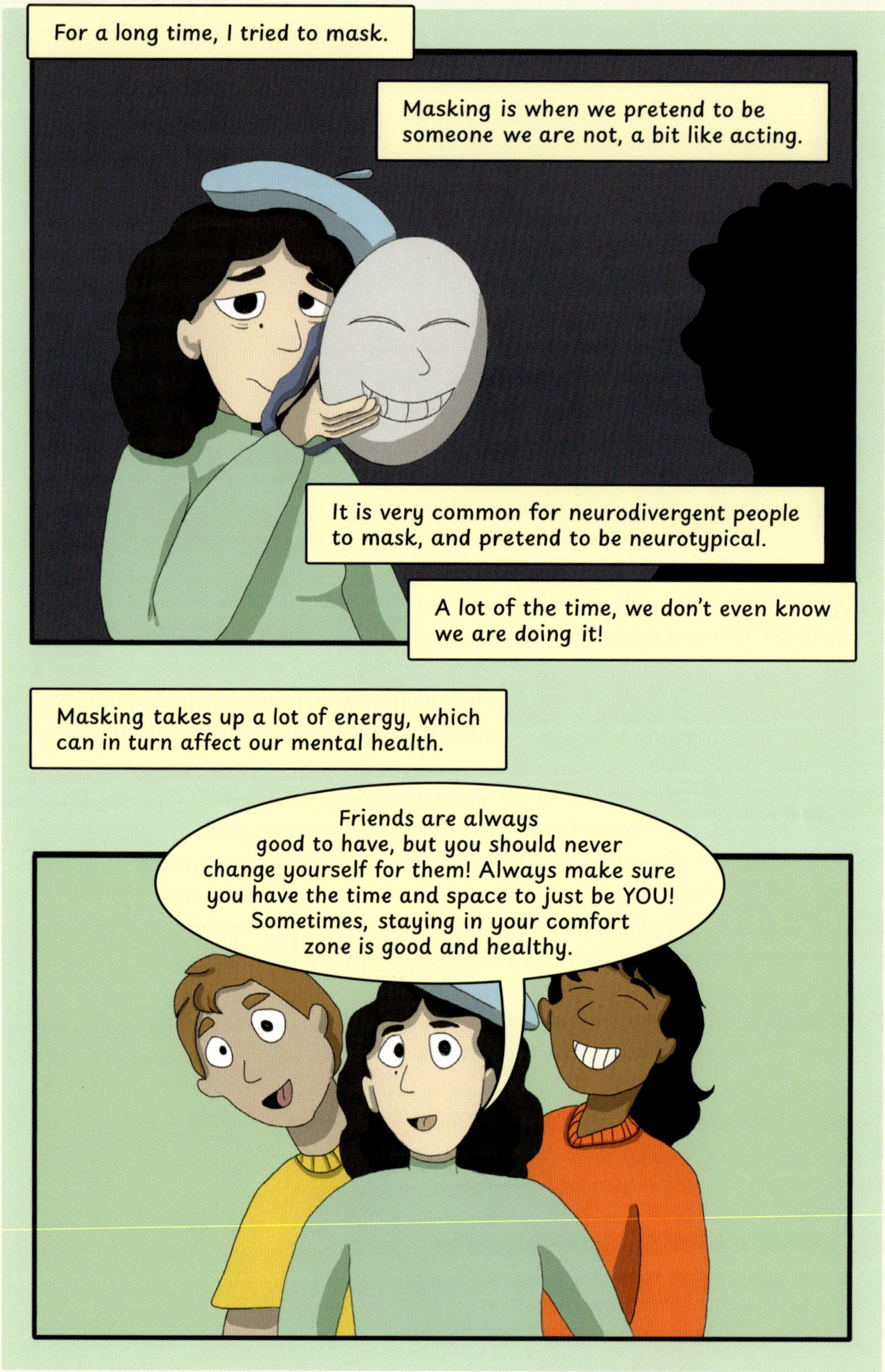

For a long time, I tried to mask.
Masking is when we pretend to be someone we are not, a bit like acting.
It is very common for neurodivergent people to mask, and pretend to be neurotypical.
A lot of the time, we don't even know we are doing it!
Masking takes up a lot of energy, which can in turn affect our mental health.
Friends are always good to have, but you should never change yourself for them! Always make sure you have the time and space to just be YOU! Sometimes, staying in your comfort zone is good and healthy.

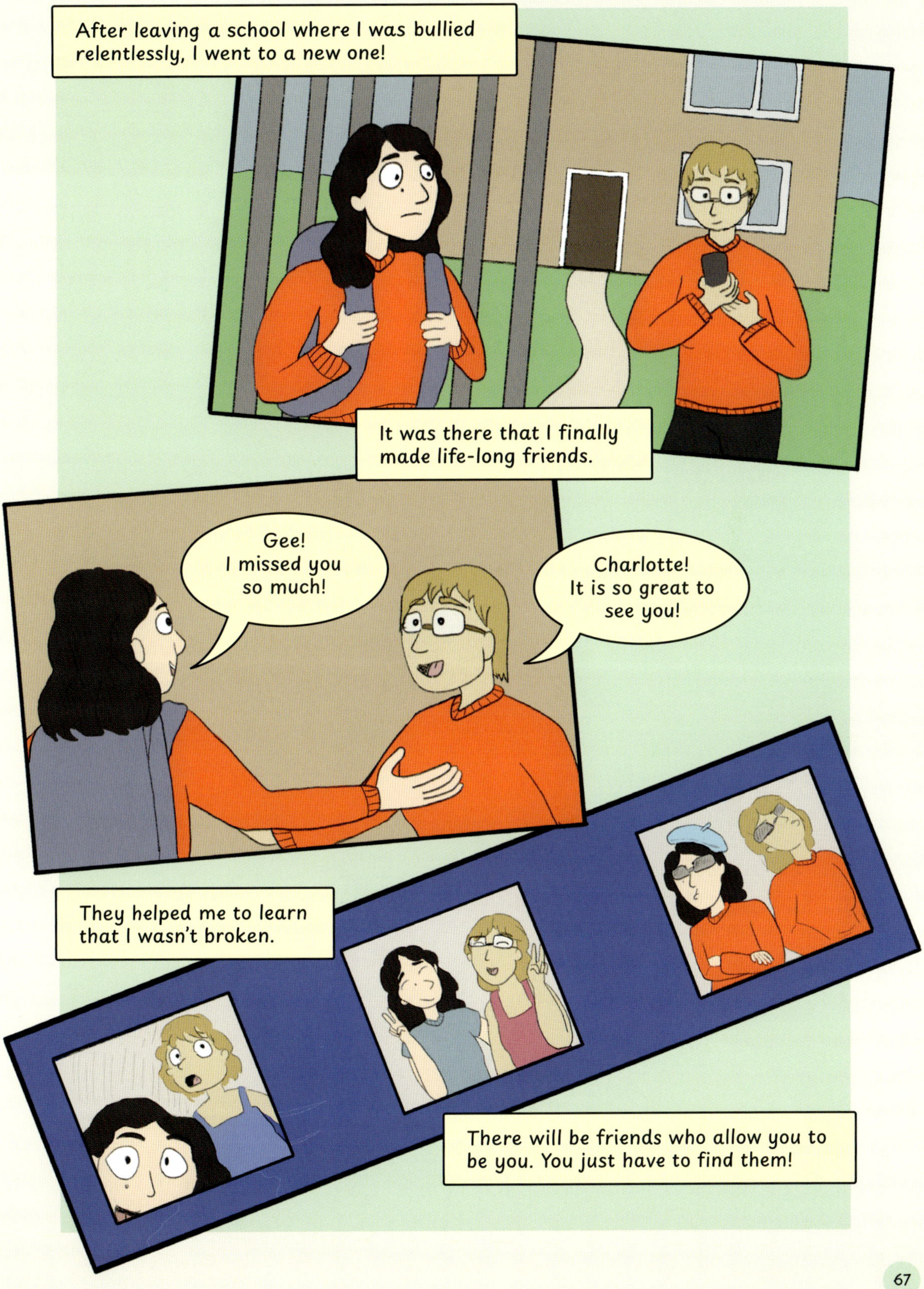
After leaving a school where I was bullied relentlessly, I went to a new one!
It was there that I finally made life-long friends.
Gee! I missed you so much!
Charlotte! It is so great to see you!
They helped me to learn that I wasn't broken.
There will be friends who allow you to be you. You just have to find them!

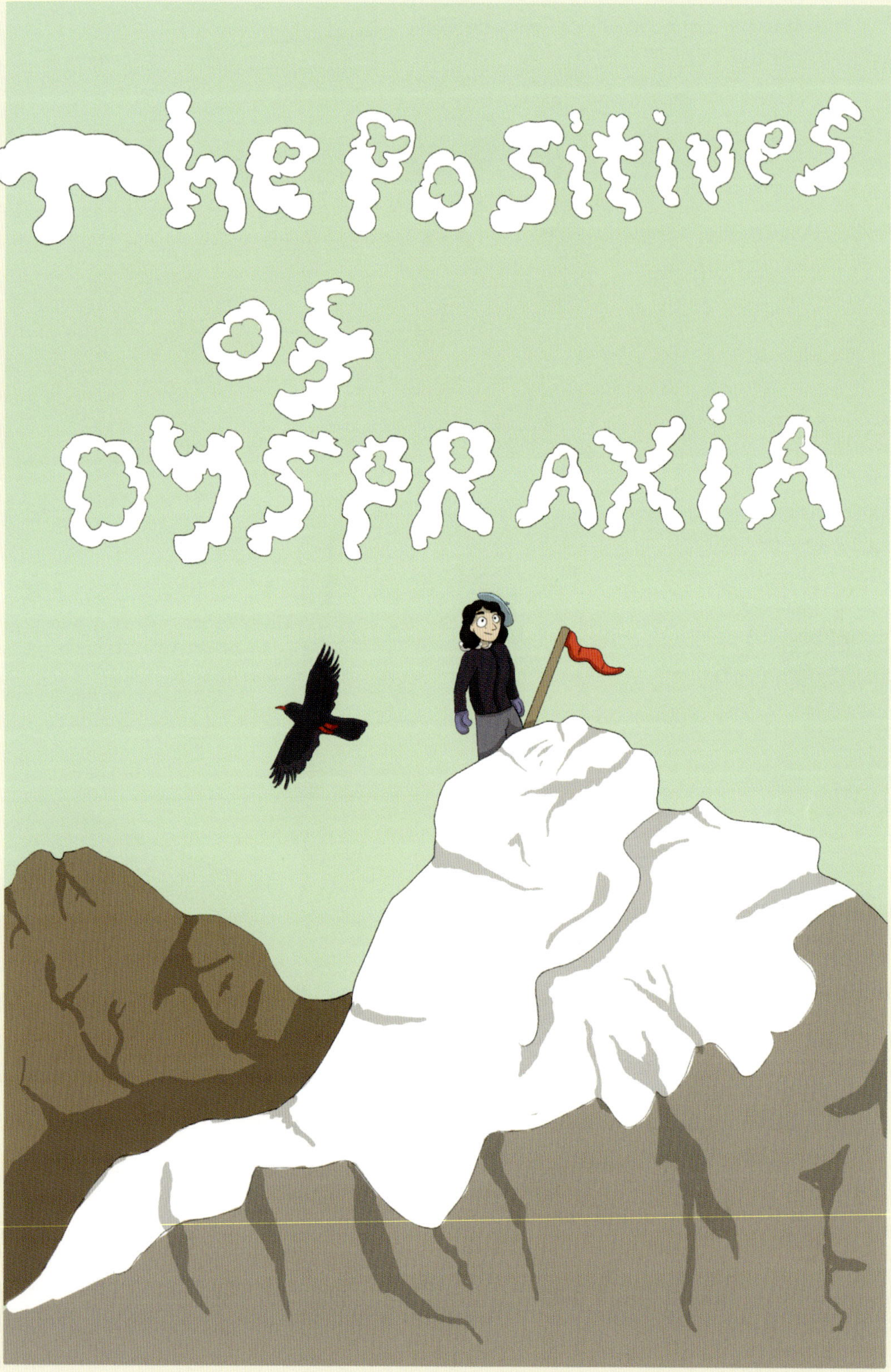
The Positives
of
DYSPRAXIA

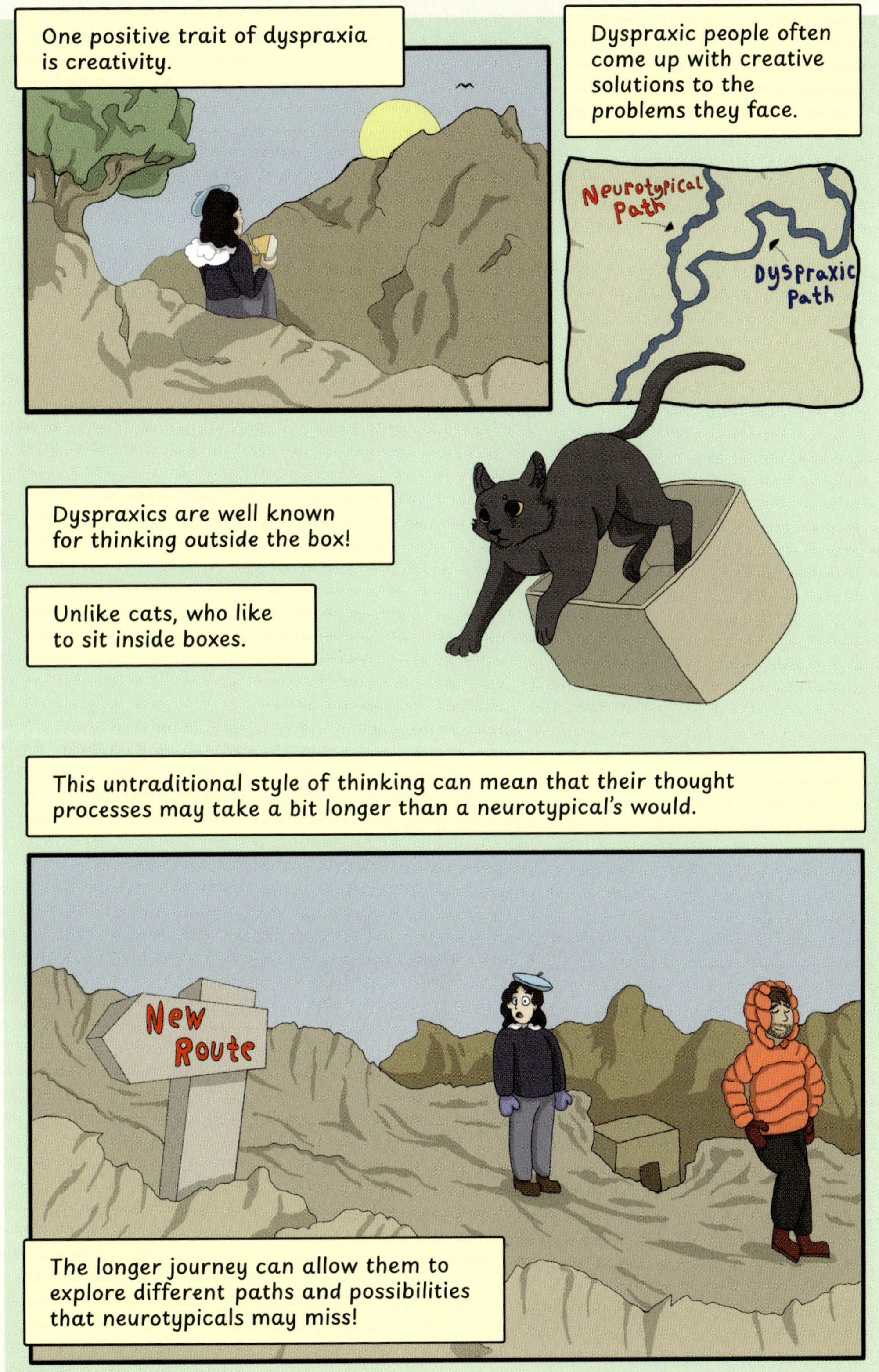
One positive trait of dyspraxia is creativity.
Dyspraxic people often come up with creative solutions to the problems they face.
Neurotypical Path
Dyspraxic Path
Dyspraxics are well known for thinking outside the box!
Unlike cats, who like to sit inside boxes.
This untraditional style of thinking can mean that their thought processes may take a bit longer than a neurotypical's would.
New Route
The longer journey can allow them to explore different paths and possibilities that neurotypicals may miss!

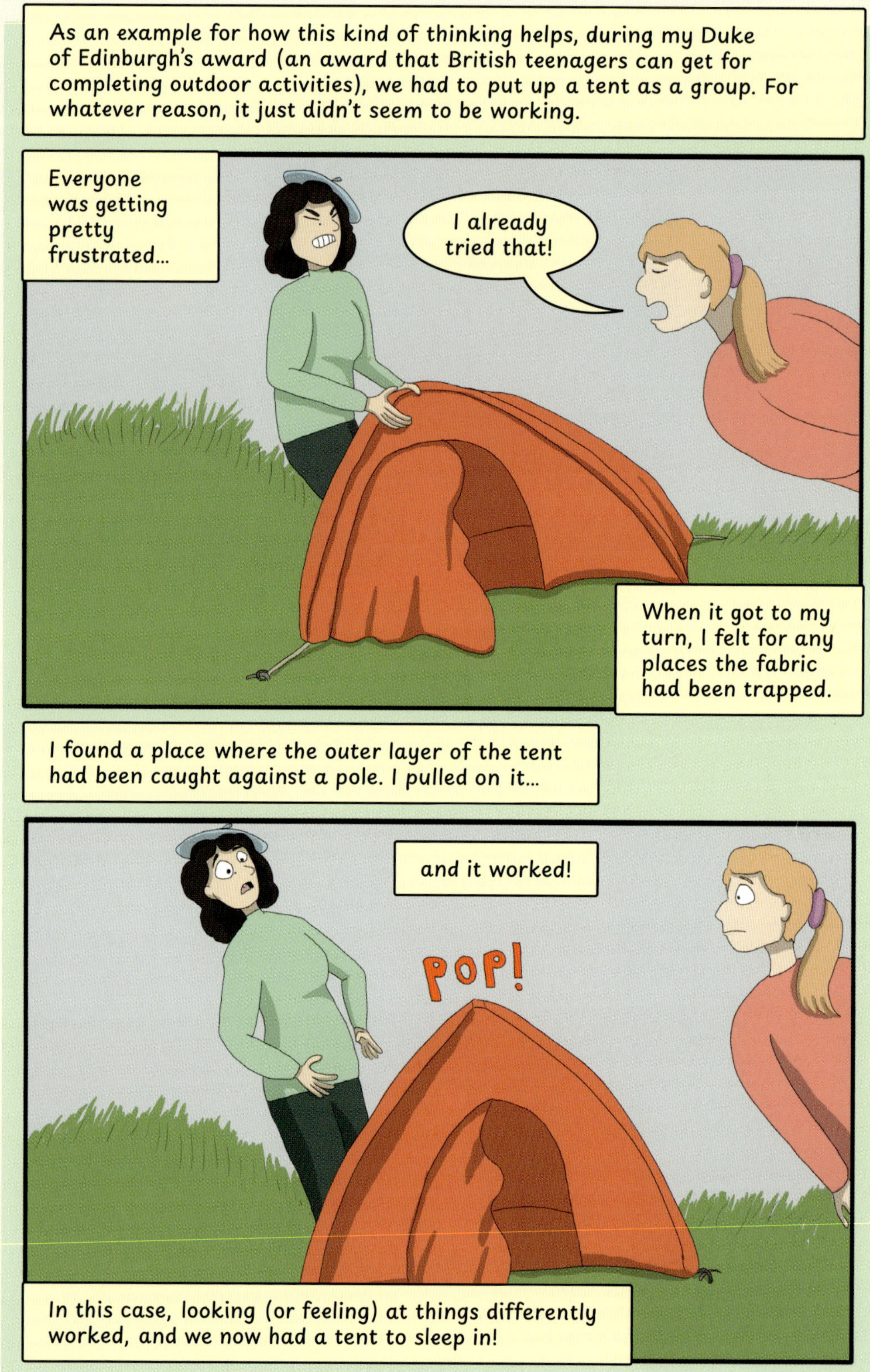
As an example for how this kind of thinking helps, during my Duke of Edinburgh's award (an award that British teenagers can get for completing outdoor activities), we had to put up a tent as a group. For whatever reason, it just didn't seem to be working.
Everyone was getting pretty frustrated...
I already tried that!
When it got to my turn, I felt for any places the fabric had been trapped.
I found a place where the outer layer of the tent had been caught against a pole. I pulled on it...
and it worked!
POP!
In this case, looking (or feeling) at things differently worked, and we now had a tent to sleep in!

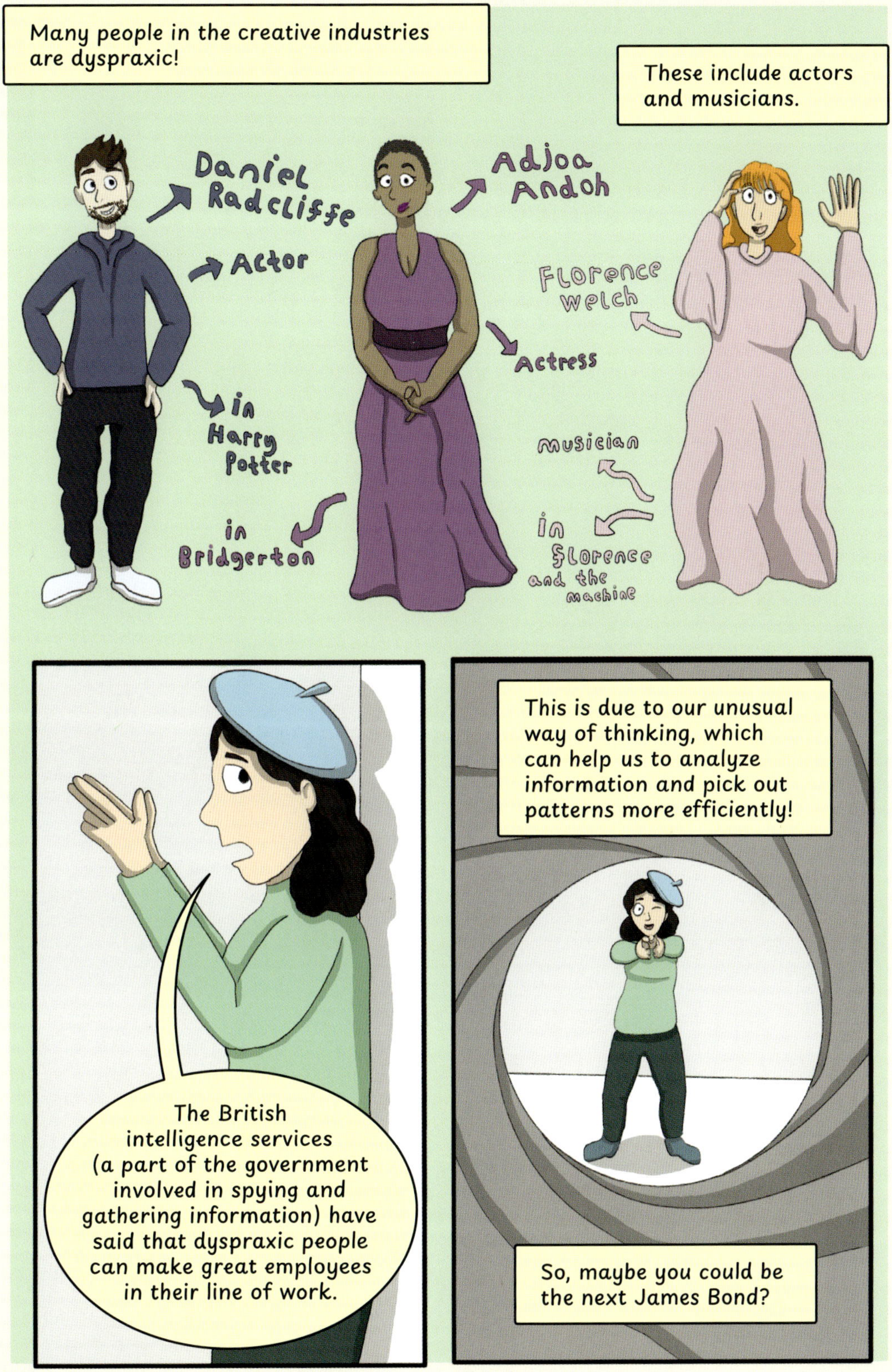

Many people in the creative industries are dyspraxic!
These include actors and musicians.
Daniel Radcliffe
Actor
in Harry Potter
Adjoa Andoh
Actress
in Bridgerton
Florence Welch
musician
in florence and the machine
The British intelligence services (a part of the government involved in spying and gathering information) have said that dyspraxic people can make great employees in their line of work.
This is due to our unusual way of thinking, which can help us to analyze information and pick out patterns more efficiently!
So, maybe you could be the next James Bond?

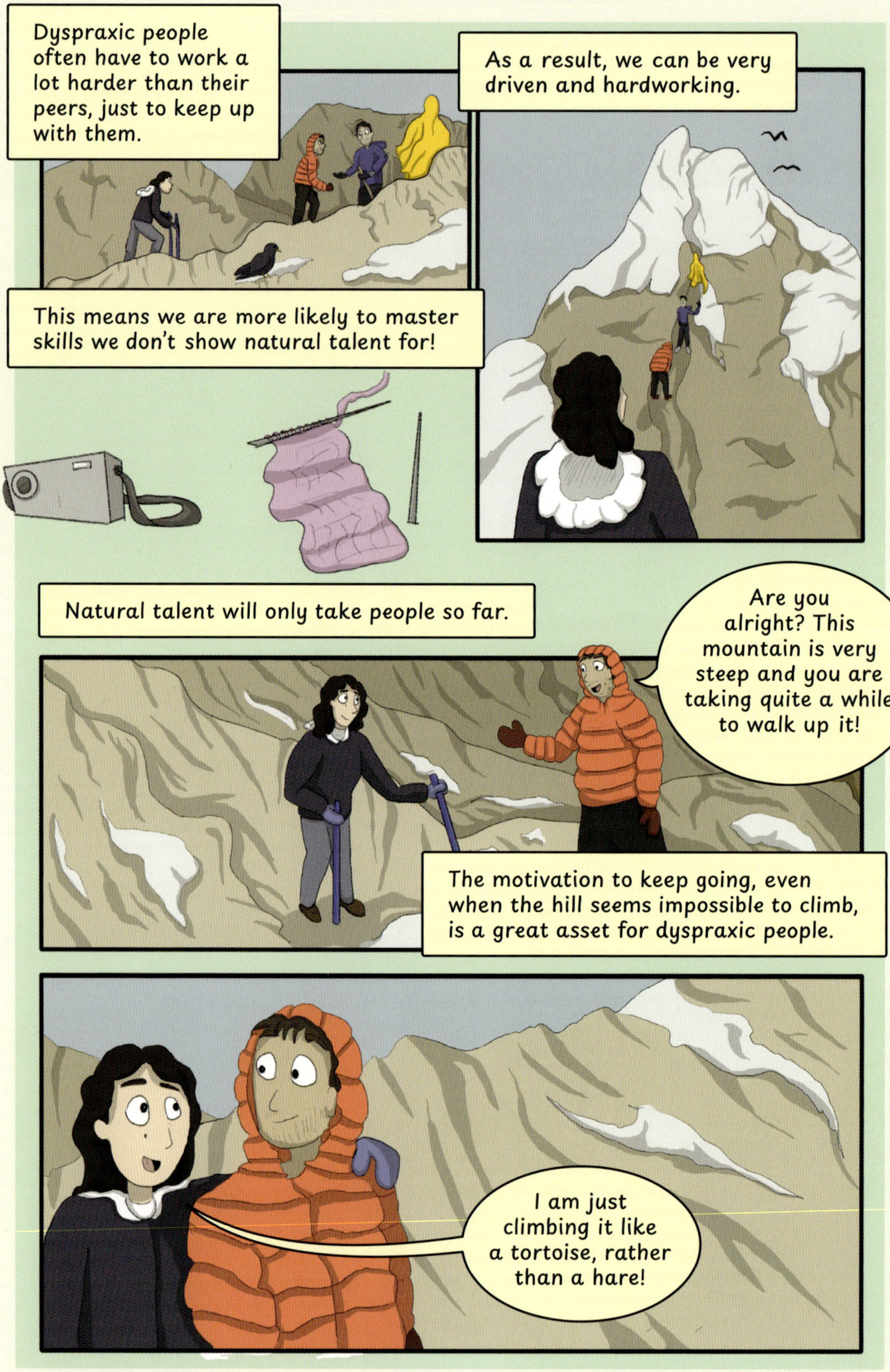
Dyspraxic people often have to work a lot harder than their peers, just to keep up with them.
This means we are more likely to master skills we don't show natural talent for!
As a result, we can be very driven and hardworking.
Natural talent will only take people so far.
Are you alright? This mountain is very steep and you are taking quite a while to walk up it!
The motivation to keep going, even when the hill seems impossible to climb, is a great asset for dyspraxic people.
I am just climbing it like a tortoise, rather than a hare!

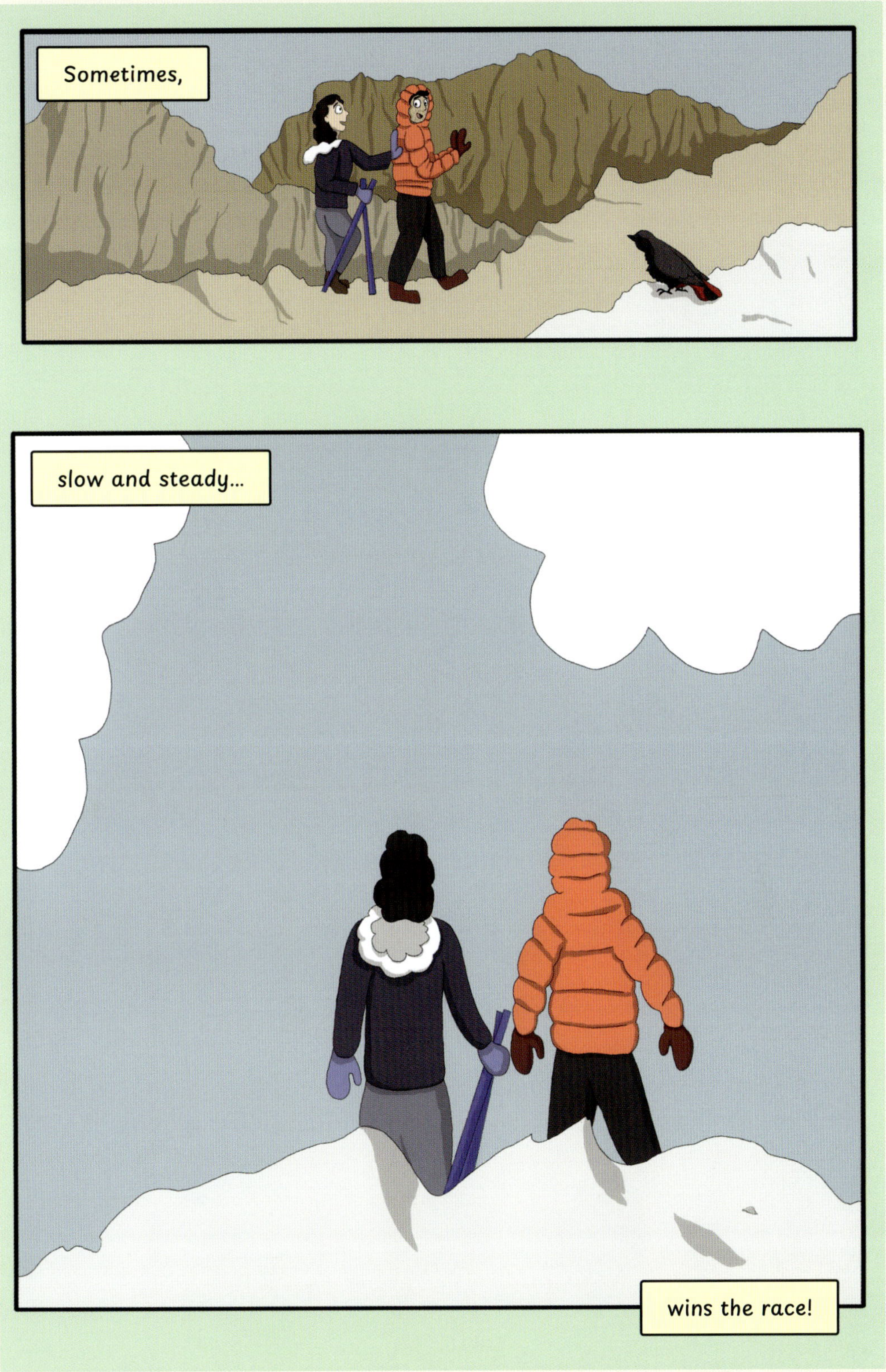
Sometimes,
slow and steady...
wins the race!

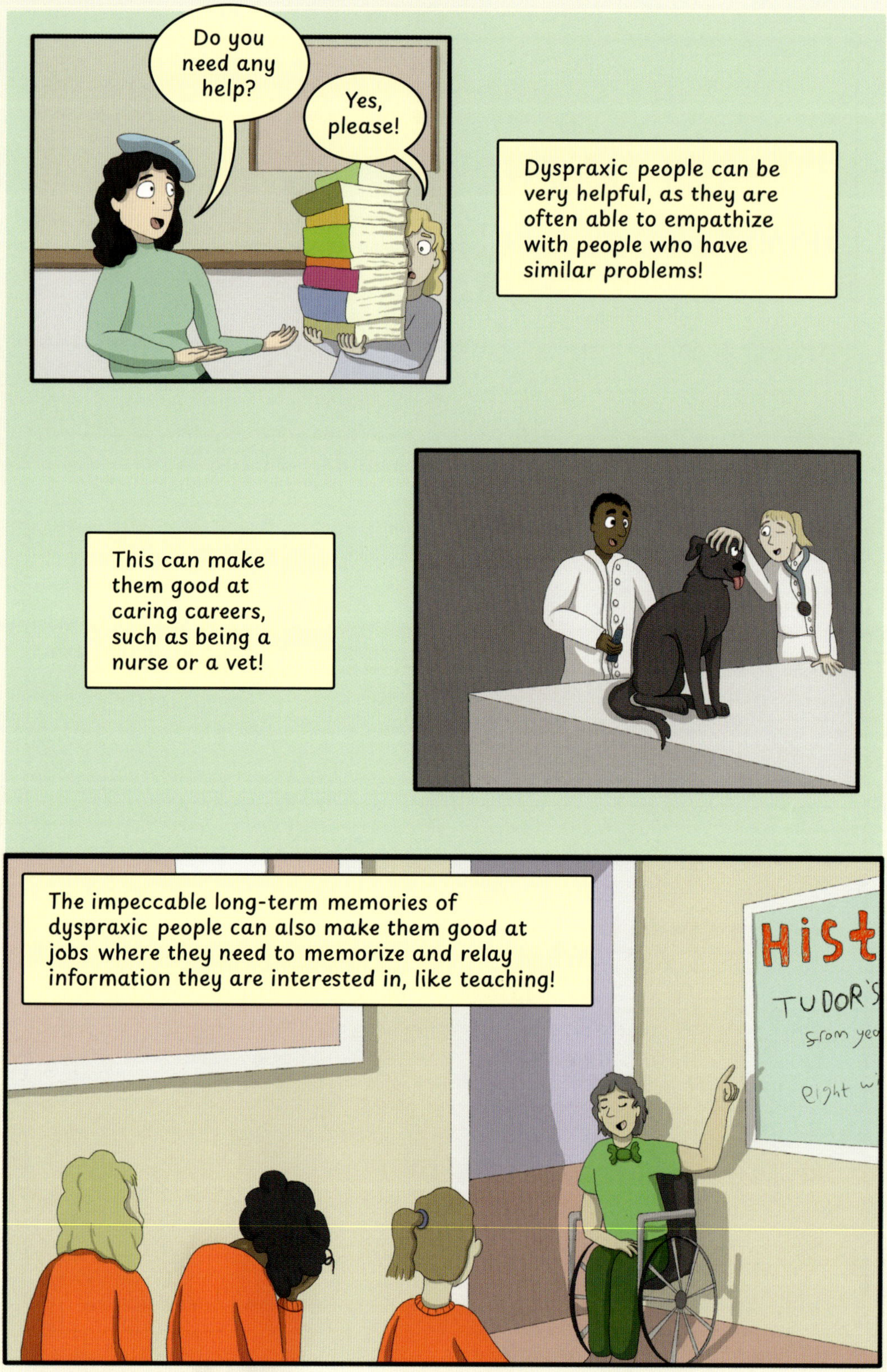
Do you need any help?
Yes, please!
Dyspraxic people can be very helpful, as they are often able to empathize with people who have similar problems!
This can make them good at caring careers, such as being a nurse or a vet!
The impeccable long-term memories of dyspraxic people can also make them good at jobs where they need to memorize and relay information they are interested in, like teaching!

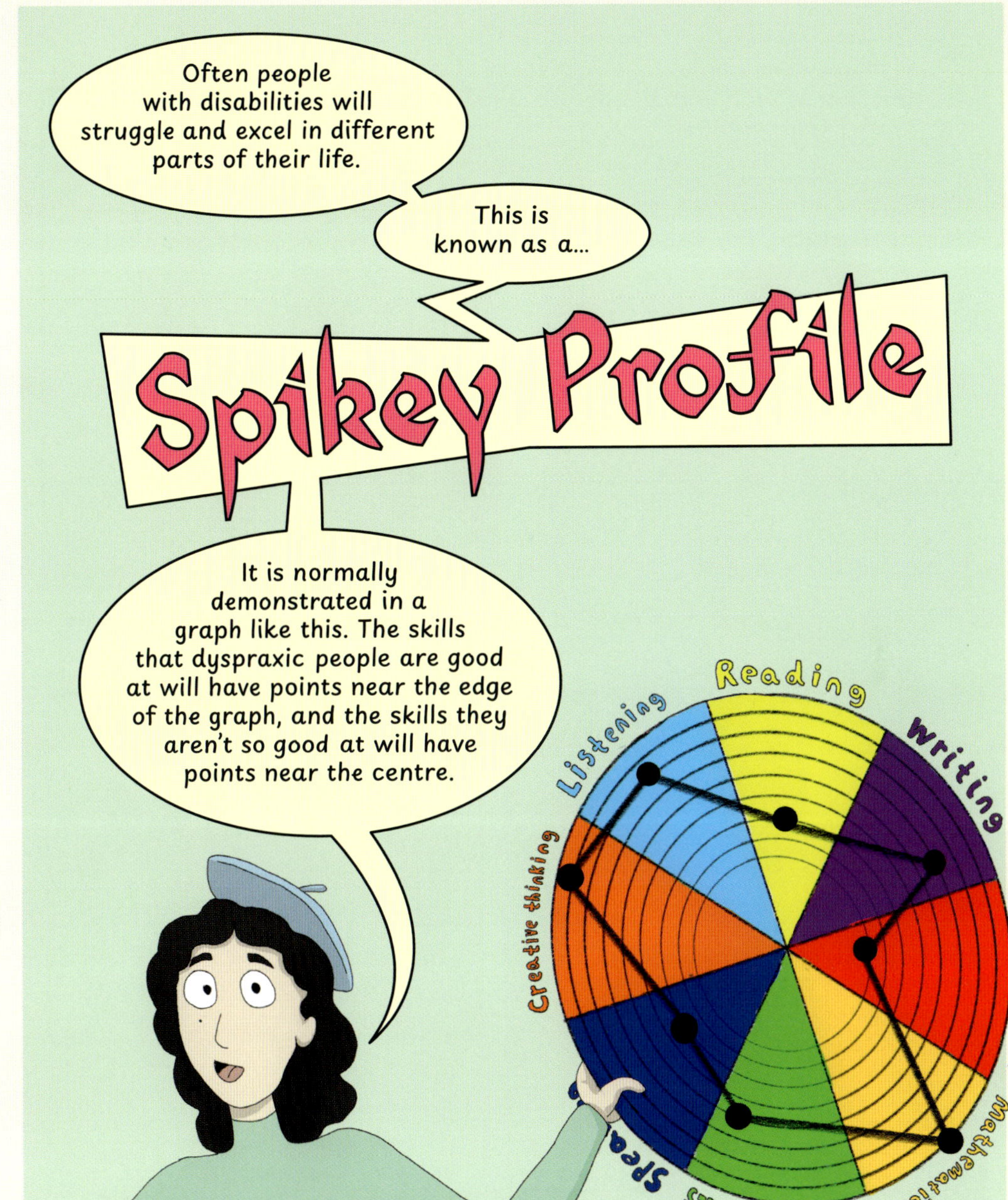

Often people with disabilities will struggle and excel in different parts of their life.
This is known as a...
Spikey Profile
It is normally demonstrated in a graph like this. The skills that dyspraxic people are good at will have points near the edge of the graph, and the skills they aren't so good at will have points near the centre.
Reading
Writing
Organization
Mathematics
Social skills
Creative thinking
Listening

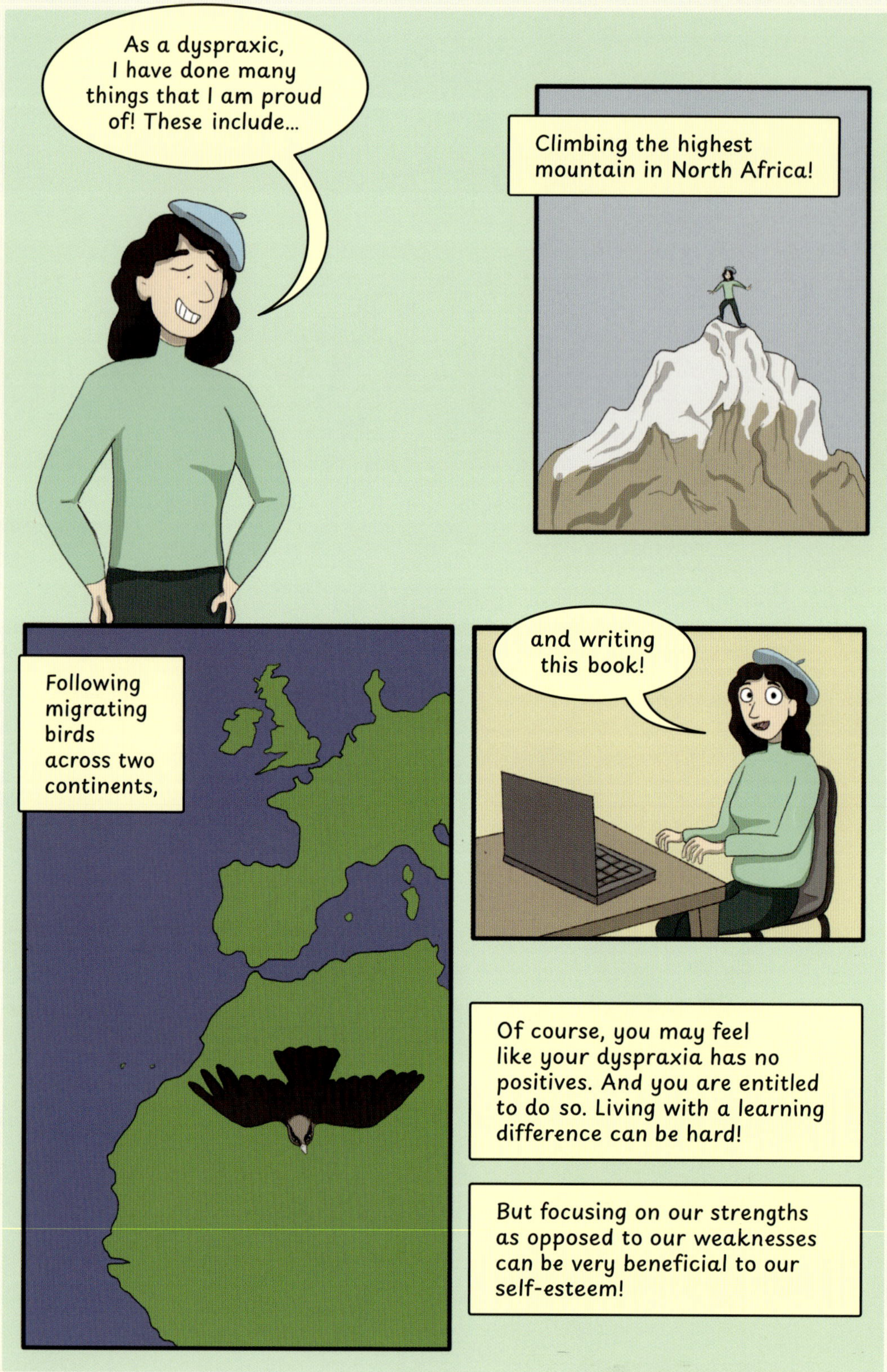
As a dyspraxic, I have done many things that I am proud of! These include...
Climbing the highest mountain in North Africa!
Following migrating birds across two continents,
and writing this book!
Of course, you may feel like your dyspraxia has no positives. And you are entitled to do so. Living with a learning difference can be hard!
But focusing on our strengths as opposed to our weaknesses can be very beneficial to our self-esteem!

Write down some positives of being dyspraxic here:

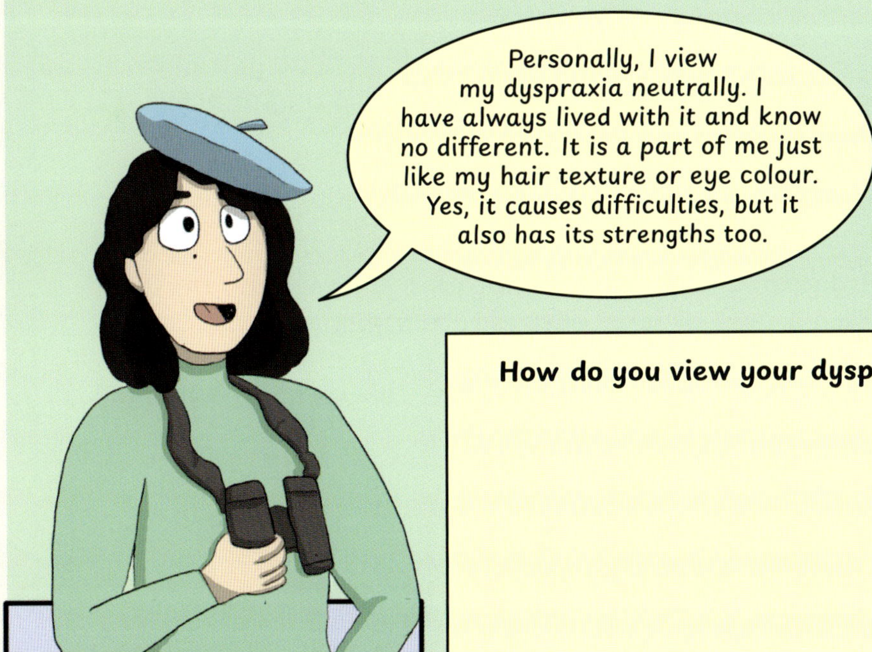
Personally, I view my dyspraxia neutrally. I have always lived with it and know no different. It is a part of me just like my hair texture or eye colour. Yes, it causes difficulties, but it also has its strengths too.

How do you view your dyspraxia?

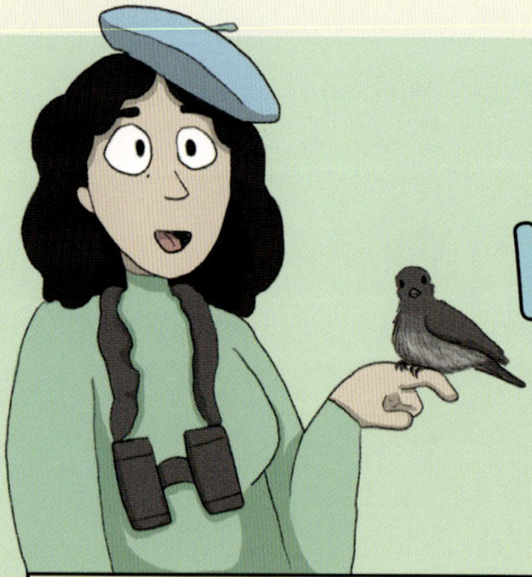

Living with Dyspraxia

Lotty's Golden List

(You may recognize some tips from the previous lists!)

- Do things in your own way. Even if it looks awkward, it is perfectly okay to do it your way and not theirs!
- Try your best! Do this for yourself so that you know that you put all of your effort in. This can improve your self-confidence!
- Always aim to get to places 15 minutes ahead of time.
- Organize yourself by writing things down and making them a part of your everyday routine.
- Focus on what you are good at. This will improve your self-esteem.
- Accept that you are different and that is okay, even a good thing!

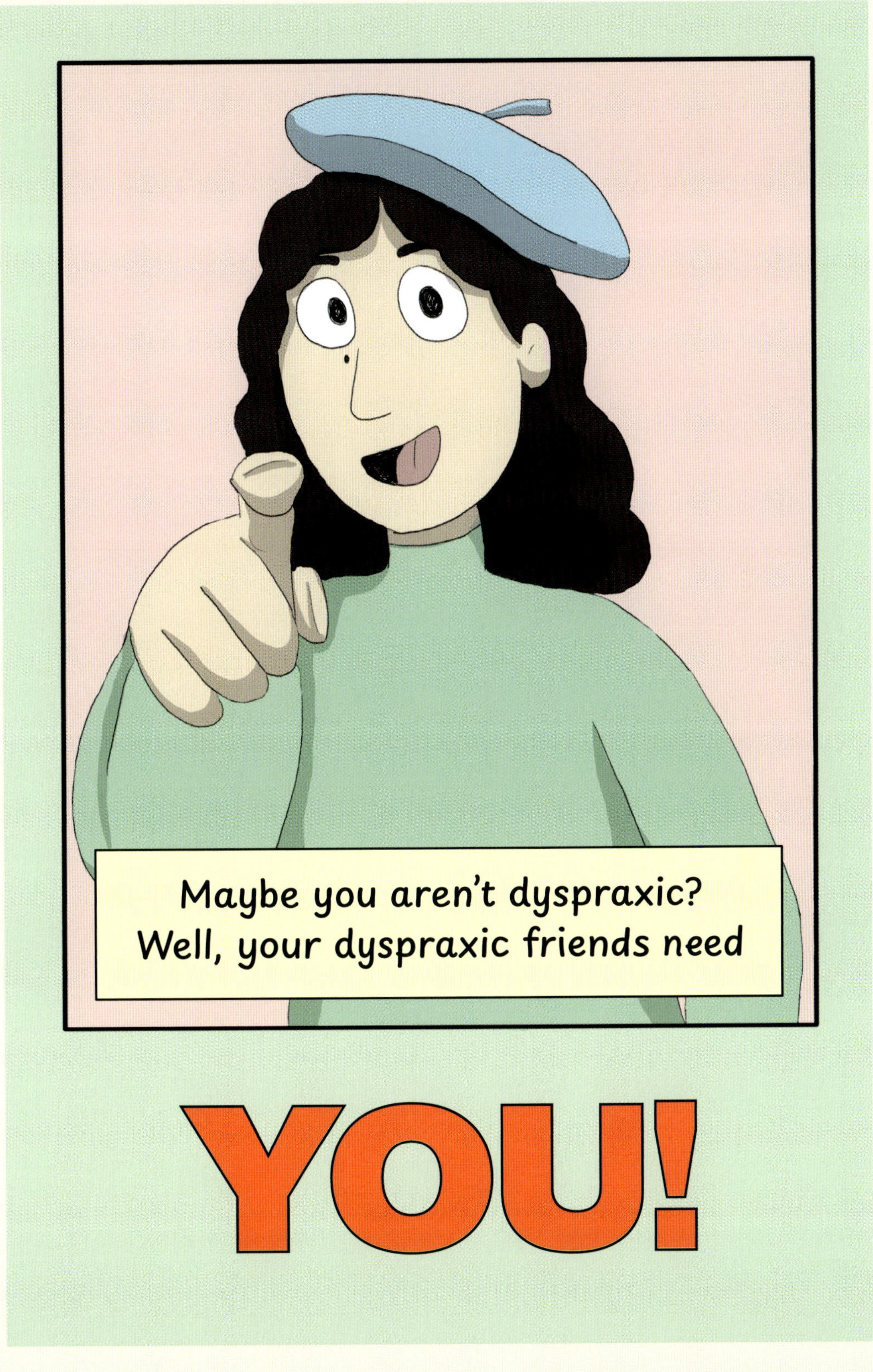
Maybe you aren't dyspraxic?
Well, your dyspraxic friends need
YOU!

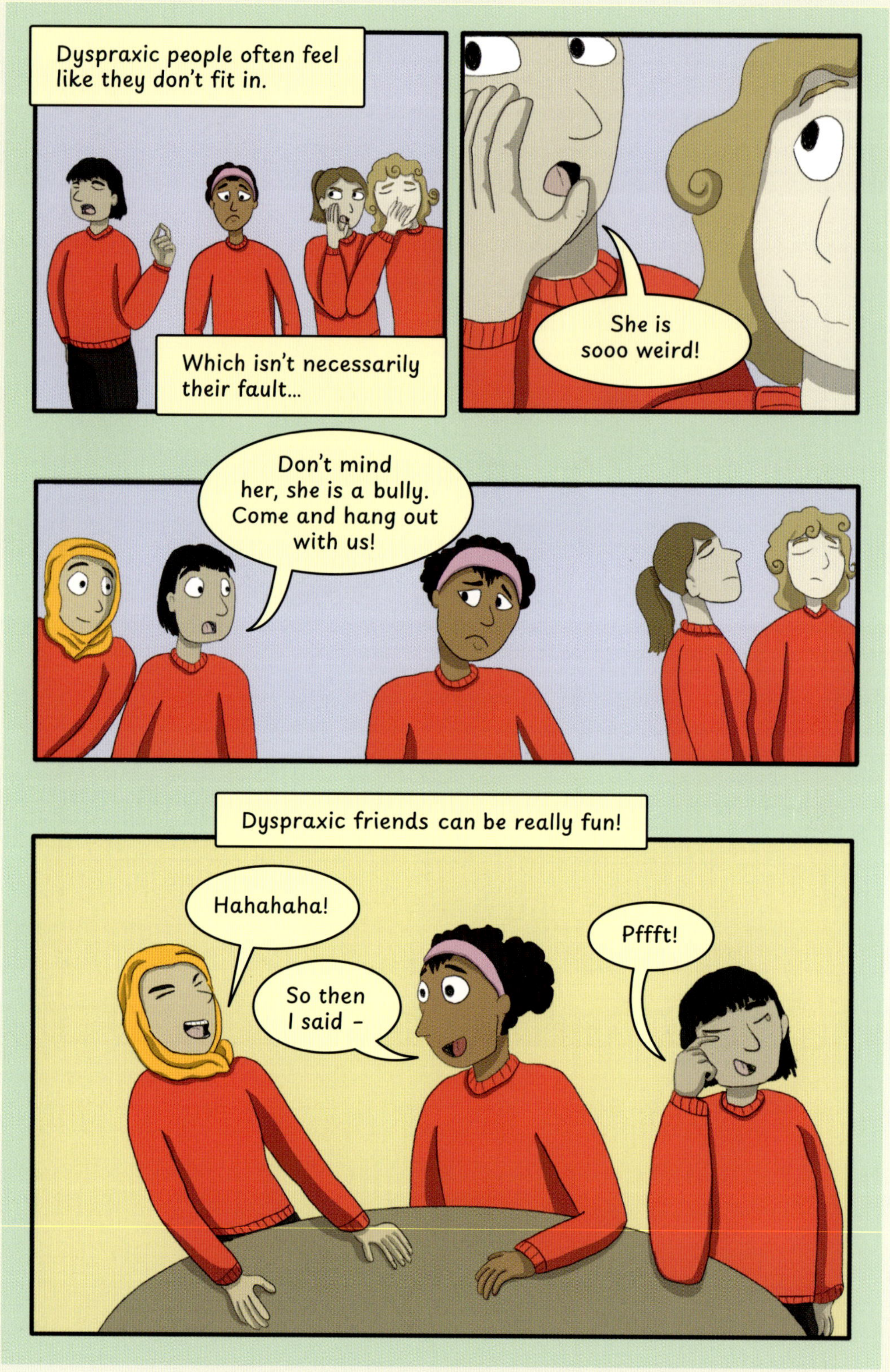
Dyspraxic people often feel like they don't fit in.
Which isn't necessarily their fault...
She is sooo weird!
Don't mind her, she is a bully. Come and hang out with us!
Dyspraxic friends can be really fun!
Hahahaha!
So then I said -
Pffft!

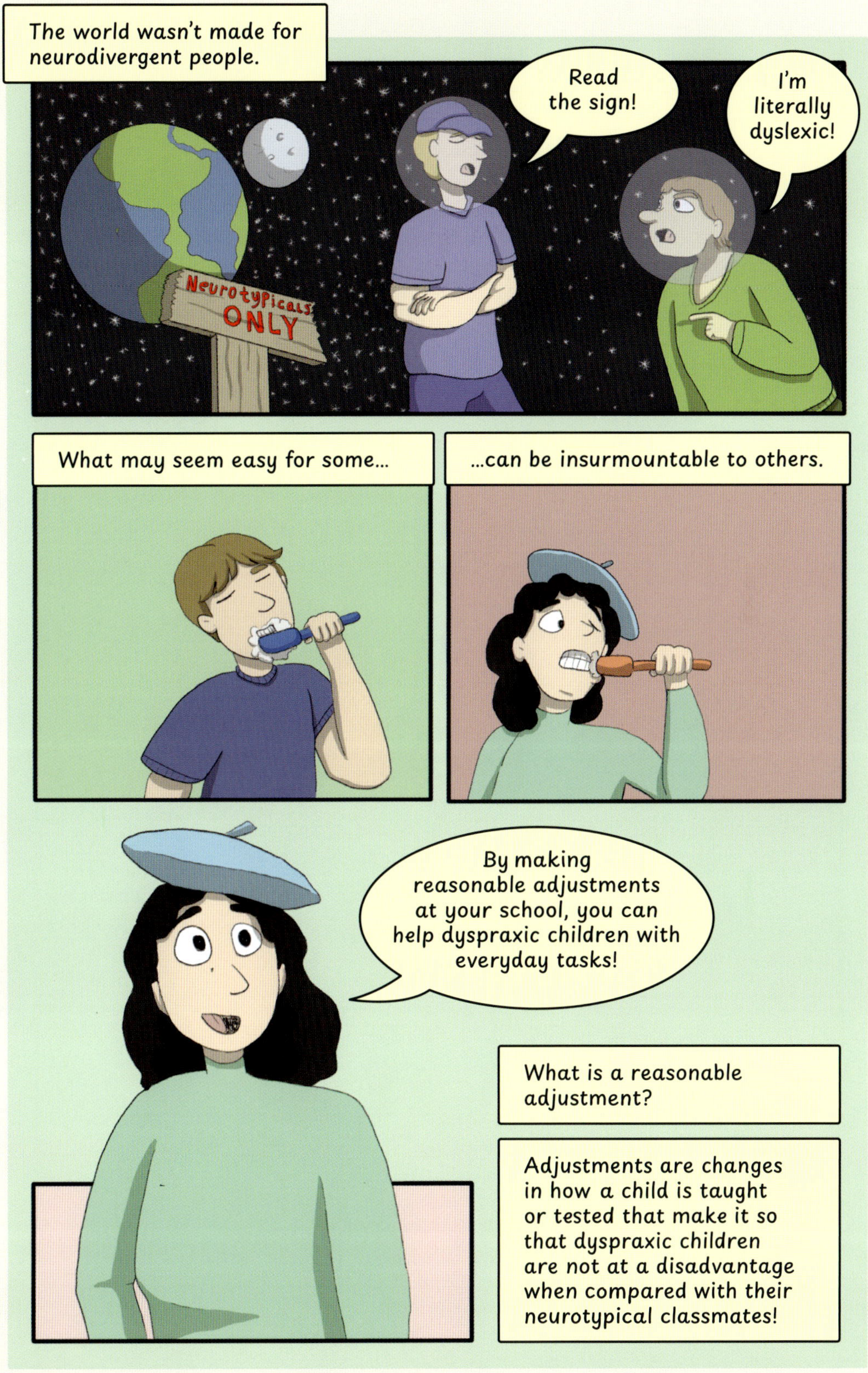
The world wasn't made for neurodivergent people.
Read the sign!
I'm literally dyslexic!
Neurotypicals ONLY
What may seem easy for some...
...can be insurmountable to others.
By making reasonable adjustments at your school, you can help dyspraxic children with everyday tasks!
What is a reasonable adjustment?
Adjustments are changes in how a child is taught or tested that make it so that dyspraxic children are not at a disadvantage when compared with their neurotypical classmates!

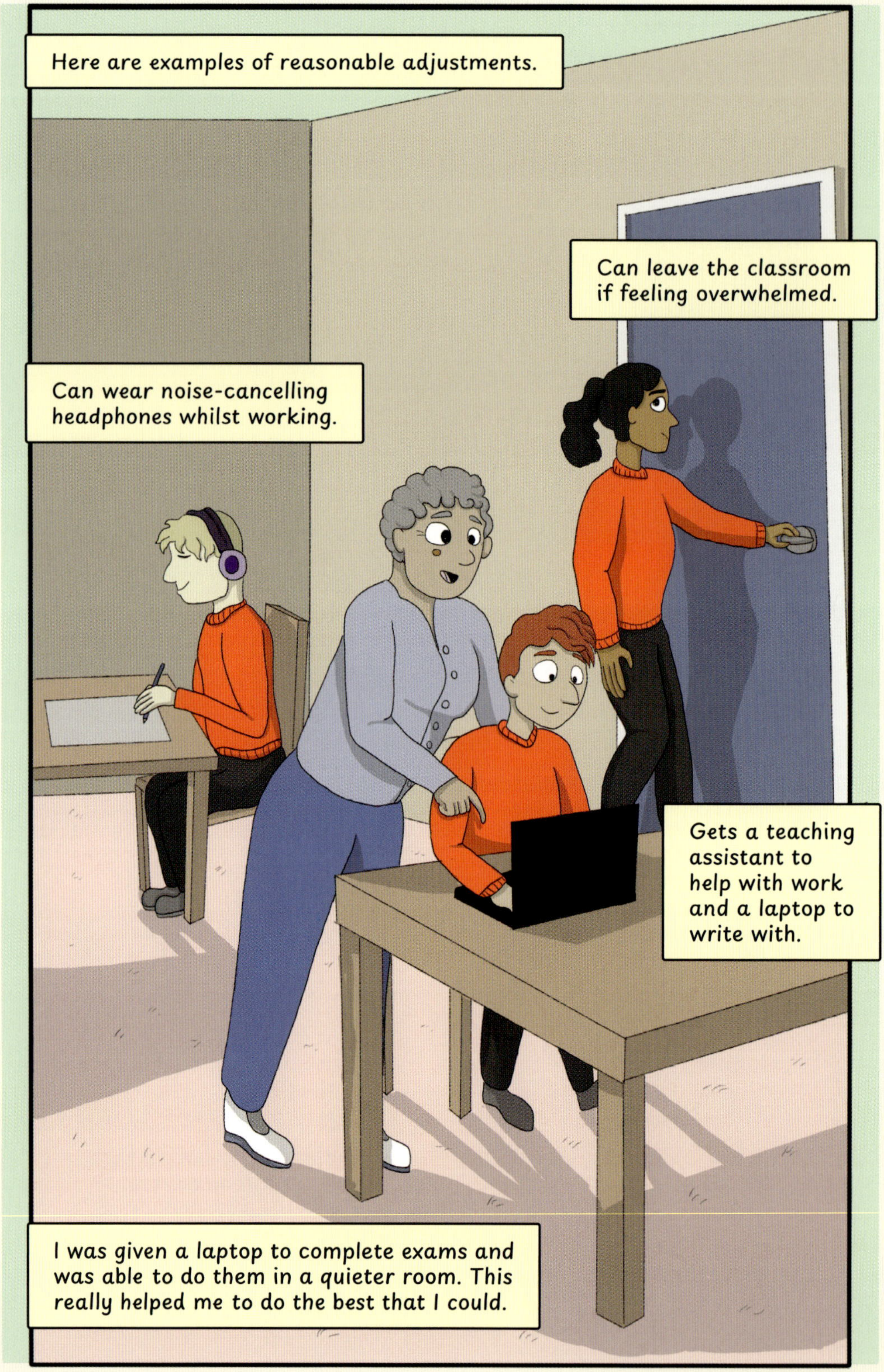
Here are examples of reasonable adjustments.
Can leave the classroom if feeling overwhelmed.
Can wear noise-cancelling headphones whilst working.
Gets a teaching assistant to help with work and a laptop to write with.
I was given a laptop to complete exams and was able to do them in a quieter room. This really helped me to do the best that I could.

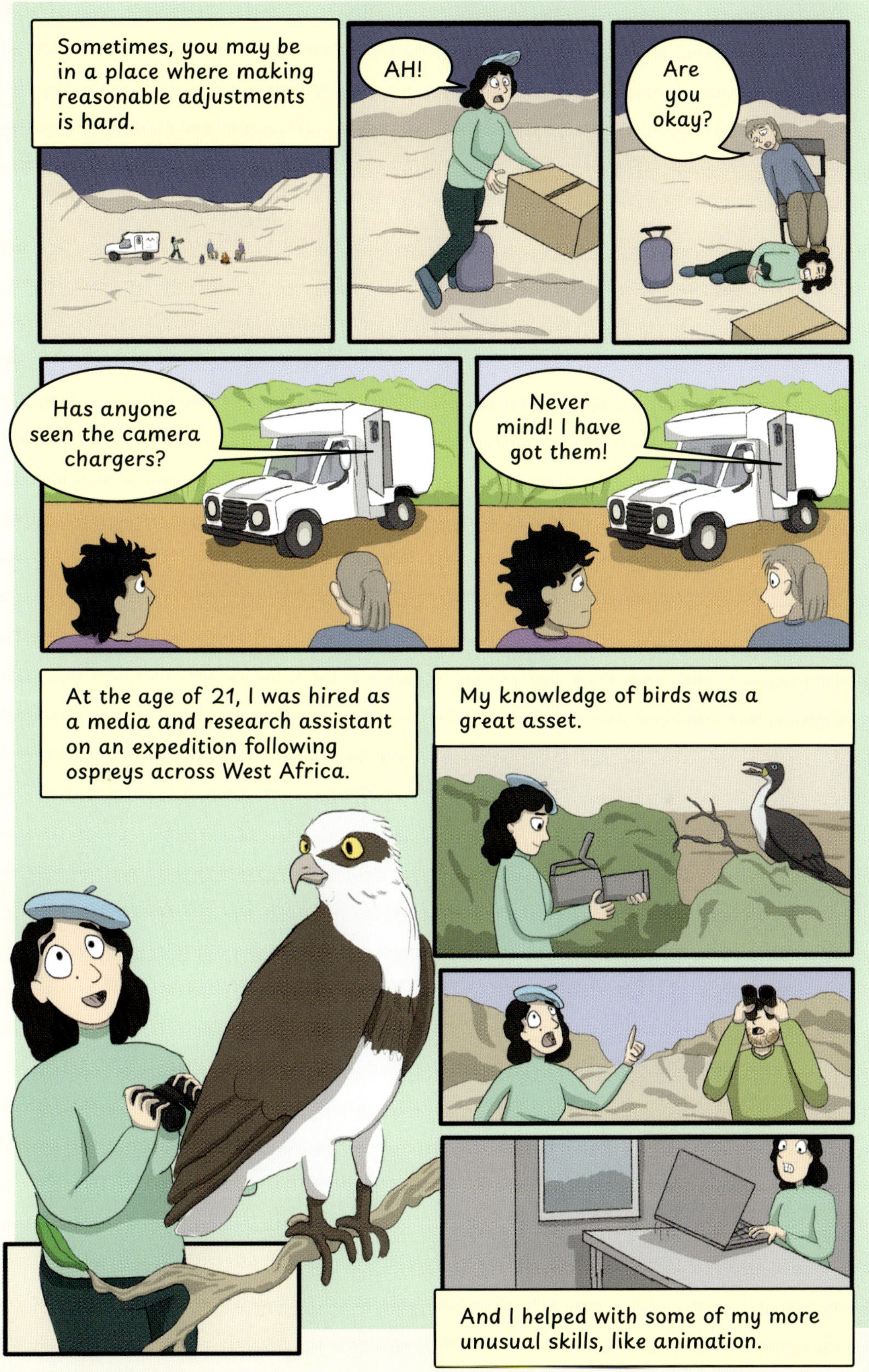
Sometimes, you may be in a place where making reasonable adjustments is hard.
AH!
Are you okay?
Has anyone seen the camera chargers?
Never mind! I have got them!
At the age of 21, I was hired as a media and research assistant on an expedition following ospreys across West Africa.
My knowledge of birds was a great asset.
And I helped with some of my more unusual skills, like animation.

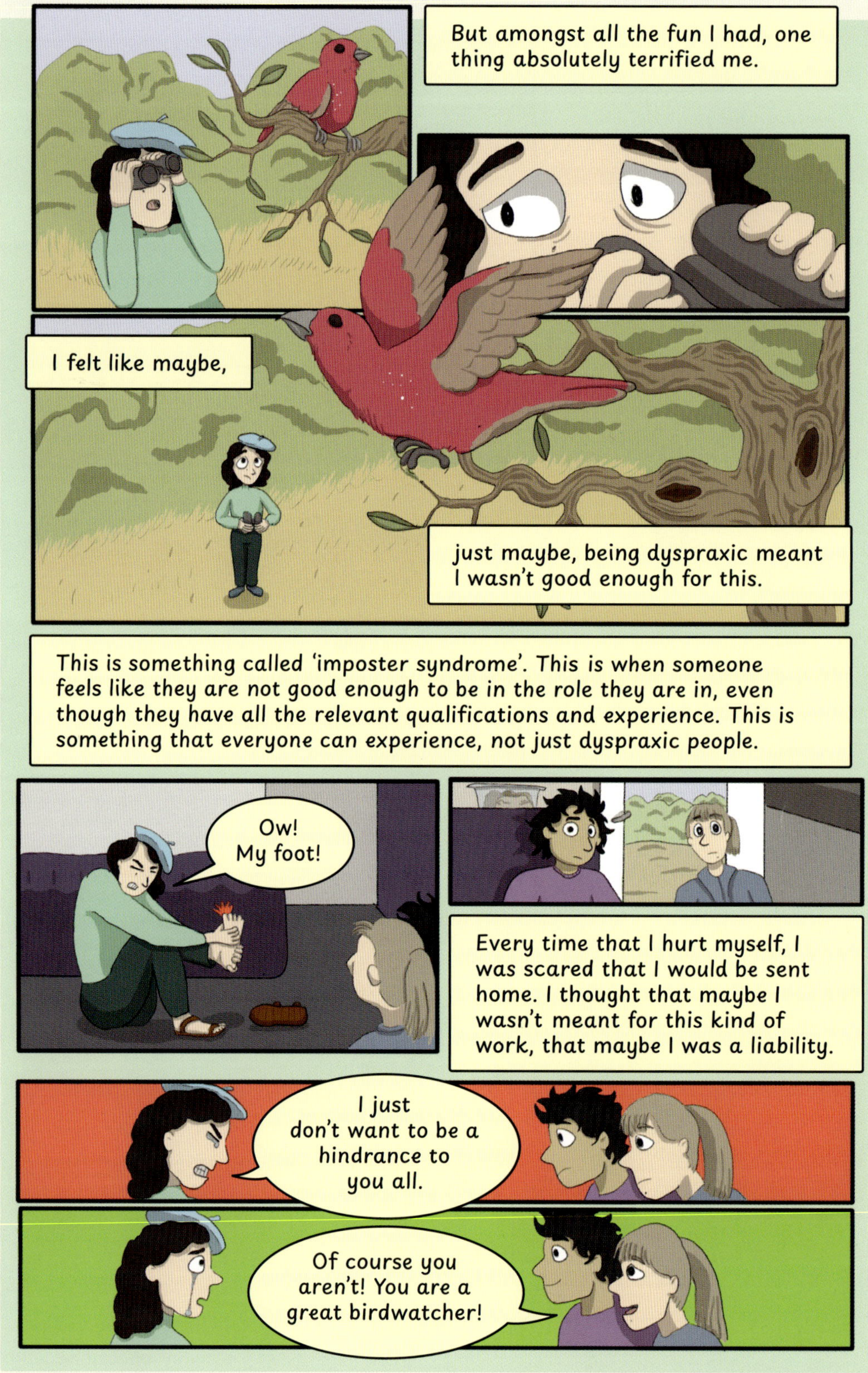

But amongst all the fun I had, one thing absolutely terrified me.
I felt like maybe,
just maybe, being dyspraxic meant I wasn't good enough for this.
This is something called 'imposter syndrome'. This is when someone feels like they are not good enough to be in the role they are in, even though they have all the relevant qualifications and experience. This is something that everyone can experience, not just dyspraxic people.
Ow! My foot!
Every time that I hurt myself, I was scared that I would be sent home. I thought that maybe I wasn't meant for this kind of work, that maybe I was a liability.
I just don't want to be a hindrance to you all.
Of course you aren't! You are a great birdwatcher!

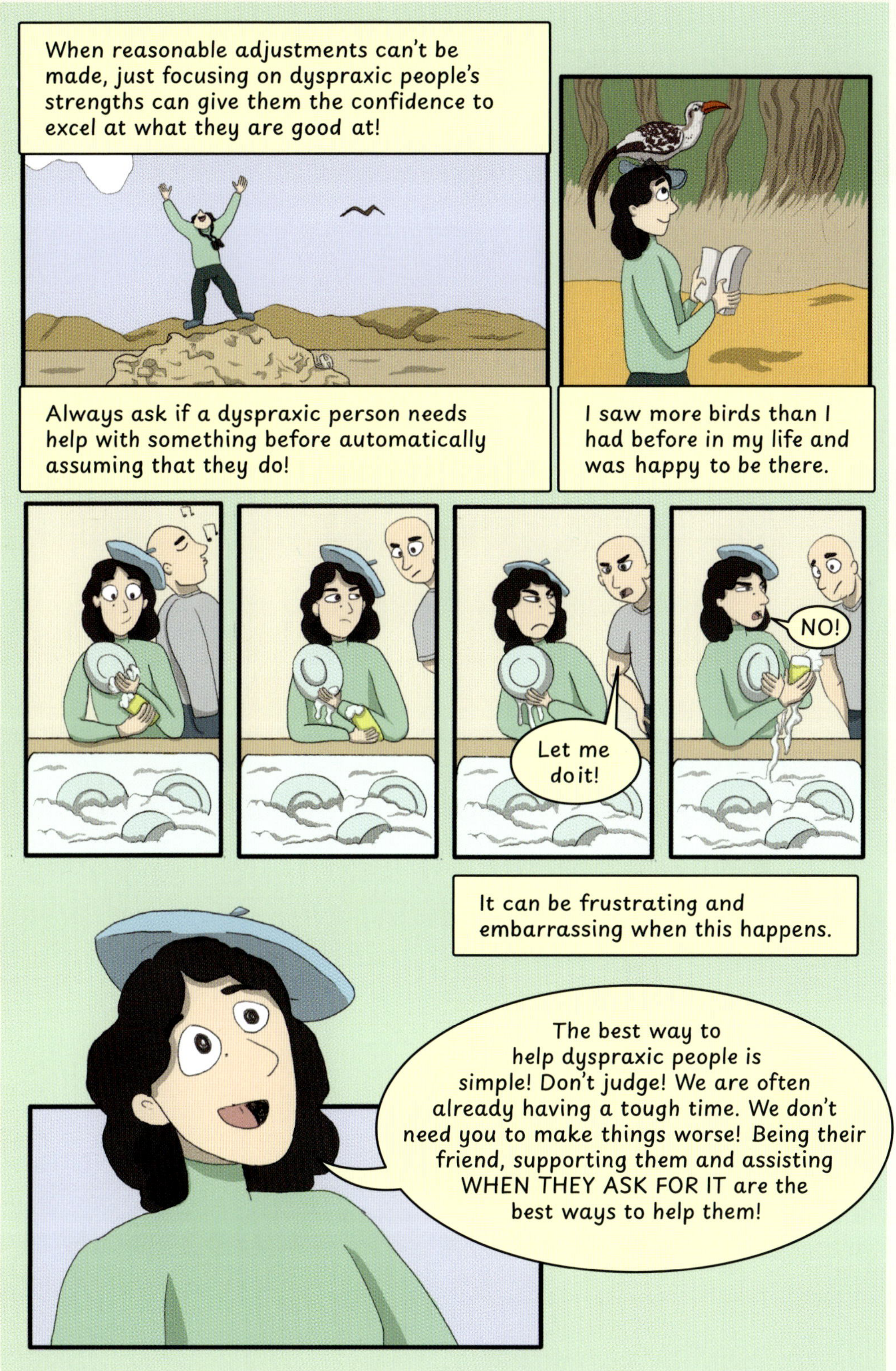

When reasonable adjustments can't be made, just focusing on dyspraxic people's strengths can give them the confidence to excel at what they are good at!
Always ask if a dyspraxic person needs help with something before automatically assuming that they do!
I saw more birds than I had before in my life and was happy to be there.
Let me do it!
NO!
It can be frustrating and embarrassing when this happens.
The best way to help dyspraxic people is simple! Don't judge! We are often already having a tough time. We don't need you to make things worse! Being their friend, supporting them and assisting WHEN THEY ASK FOR IT are the best ways to help them!

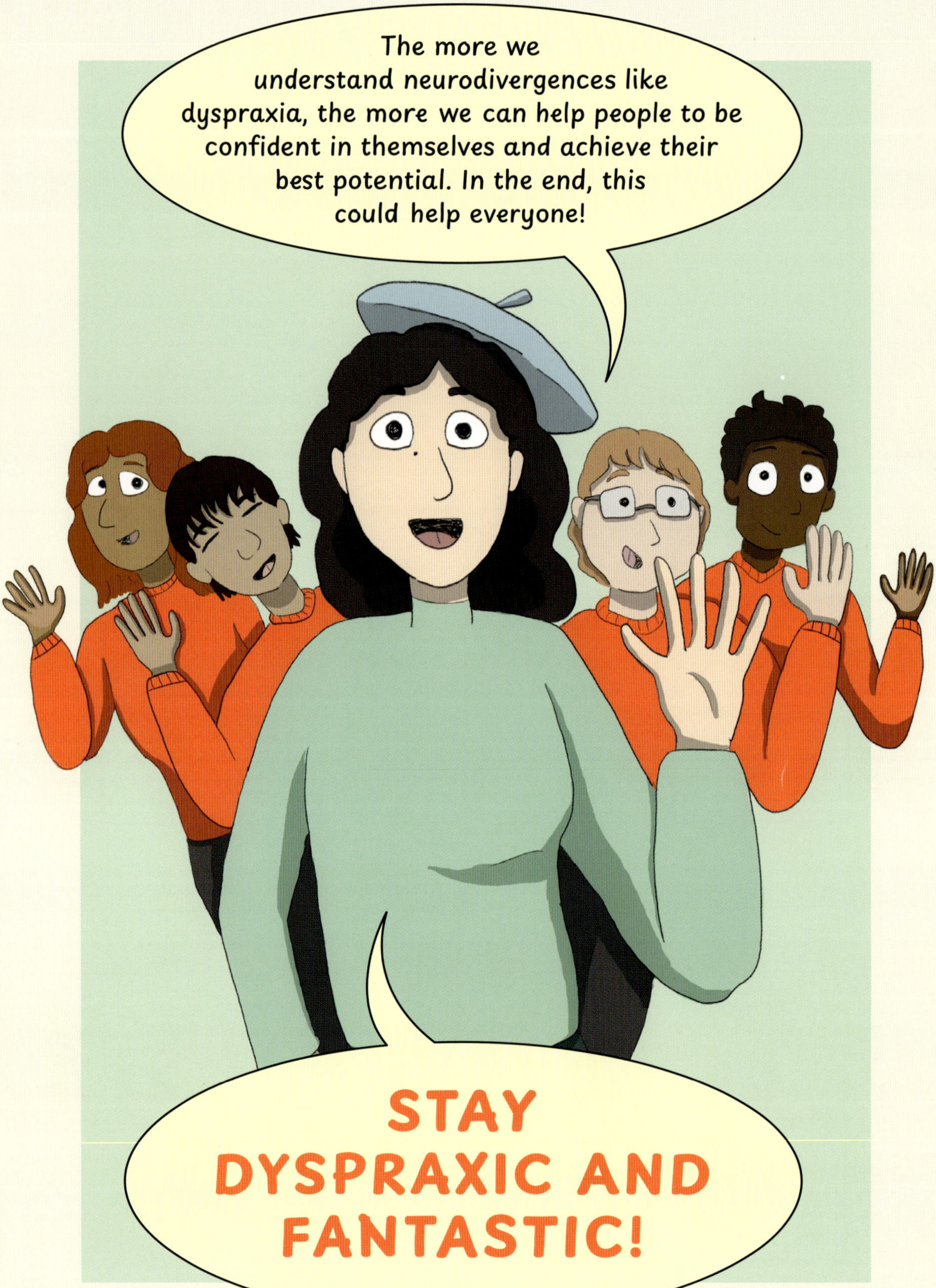
The more we understand neurodivergences like dyspraxia, the more we can help people to be confident in themselves and achieve their best potential. In the end, this could help everyone!
STAY DYSPRAXIC AND FANTASTIC!